The Vital Blend

"Five Ways to Dramatically Improve Your Health"

By Anthony Vita

Table of Contents

CHAPTER ONE
We Are All Being Poisoned!

"Today, the foods we eat are mostly PRODUCTS made and sold by CORPORATIONS. Like any other product a corporation sells, they are driven by certain principles to be successful; manufacture their products as cheaply as possible, convince customers they need it and then advertise it to them endlessly."

We are all being POISONED! Doesn't this sound like a shocking way to begin a book about health? You may think I'm over-exaggerating by making such a **bold** statement. However, let's see if you still feel the same after I've had some time to present you with evidence that supports my claim.

So, let's start again...

I have some good news and some bad news for you...

The BAD news is that we are all being poisoned.

The GOOD news is that there is still something we can do about it before it's too late.

You see, I was being poisoned too; my health was suffering as a result and then I discovered a way to reverse it. Once I realized the direct link between the food I was eating, the weight I had gained and how badly I was feeling, my health turned around for the better. *Whether your goal is to lose weight, fight a disease or improve your overall health, just know it is possible to PREVENT, FIGHT and REVERSE most of the health issues we face today, simply by changing what we eat.*

When it comes to food, much of what you'll find in grocery stores or restaurants today did not even exist 50-100 years ago. The most successful civilizations on the planet survived and THRIVED in large numbers over many thousands of years and across vast distances not by ordering takeout or having dinner handed to them at a drive-thru window.

Today, the foods we eat are mostly PRODUCTS made and sold by CORPORATIONS. Like any other product a corporation sells, they are driven by certain principles to be successful; manufacture their products as cheaply as possible, convince customers they need it and then advertise it to them ENDLESSLY.

When it comes to the production of our food this means companies prefer to use CHEMICALS instead of real ingredients to cut costs. A good example is Azodicarbonamide, a chemical used to improve the elasticity of dough and common in many fast food sandwiches or grocery store breads. Surprisingly, this same chemical is ALSO found in synthetic leather and rubber products such as yoga mats and shoes. Azodicarbonamide has been linked to serious health issues from asthma to cancer.

Another example would be the use of Yellow #6, a chemical dye used as coloring in foods like macaroni & cheese and snack chips. Not only are these dyes known carcinogens, they have also been linked to hyperactivity, skin rashes and migraines in children.

Food manufacturers make use of these chemicals TO SAVE MONEY so they don't have to spend it on real, natural ingredients. While big corporations are saving money, the real cost is to OUR health.

No wonder most of the population are suffering with health issues at epidemic rates. Imagine eating a sandwich containing one chemical and then drinking a soda with yet another. These toxic "cocktails" are mixing inside our bodies EVERY day and ravaging our health. It happened to me, it can happen to you and likely to someone you care very much about, such as a close friend, parent or child.

MY DISCOVERY

For nearly three years I had been working in business sales at a multinational, Fortune 50 company in Nashville and the corporate way of life was beginning to take its toll on my health. My demanding job often meant little time for eating and poor decisions when I did.

During that time I used every single one of my allotted days set aside for sickness and personal time to deal with health issues such as head colds, stomach bugs, headaches, fevers, sore throats, strep throat and brain fog. Seeing a doctor provided little help, as he only prescribed medications that relieved my symptoms but did not address the root CAUSE of my illnesses.

It wasn't until a visit from one of my best friends, Chris, that I decided it was time to step back and reevaluate everything I was eating and why. Chris had been struggling with symptoms of chronic fatigue, fibromyalgia and experiencing musculo-skeletal type pain in his chest, neck and sides. After consulting with numerous doctors and having thousands of dollars billed to his insurance company for MRIs and other tests, not a single one was able to determine what CAUSED his pain. All the doctors wanted to do was bill for more tests. Chris had enough of this, did his own research and shifted his diet to one that incorporated more real, naturally grown foods and less packaged, processed ones. I could see personally how he both looked and felt better than he had in years.

You've heard the old saying: "You are what you eat". That means I was closer to General Tso than a celery stick. If I had one major take away after watching what Chris did to heal himself – I needed to stop eating heavily processed, "junk" foods and eat more FRUITS and GREENS. If I was going to get my health back on track I had to quickly get over my reluctance to eat vegetables.

You see, at the restaurant, I was the one passing on the FREE salad that came with the meal. At the Chinese buffet, I was the guy who goes straight for the fried foods like General's chicken, fried rice, and sweet and sour pork. Sure, I would grab a couple of broccoli spears in good faith, but they were still on my plate when the waiter walked it away.

If I was going to start eating vegetables, I had to come up with something radical (for me anyway) to make it easy and tasty at the same time. I FINALLY realized the solution to my dilemma when I discovered "green smoothies".

While smoothies are beverages prepared in a blender using a mixture of fruit and ice, a "green smoothie" is one that includes green vegetables. I learned you could combine both fruits AND vegetables into a homemade drink using a blender that not only tasted terrific but supplied a generous, healthy, "shot" of nutrition as well.

Now HERE was something I could get behind. If I could gain the benefits of vegetables by DRINKING them without wanting to throw up, we may have a deal!

Not already owning a blender, I picked up a Nutribullet. It's a small, inexpensive yet powerful and highly portable blender specially designed for pulverizing everything from fruits and vegetables to nuts and seeds. Once I began cutting out the junk food and added a green smoothie to my day, the results were UNDENIABLE. Not only did I lose 50lbs and drop three pant sizes over the course of a year, but EVERY SINGLE health problem I struggled with earlier was GONE and hasn't returned, not even a runny nose.

I was so impressed with how quickly I shed pounds AND felt better that I just had to learn MORE. What was happening that caused me to lose weight? Why do certain foods make you feel sick while others make you feel remarkable? Then, I started wondering about OTHER changes I could make to feel even BETTER.

I did a tremendous amount of research over many months by reading books, news articles, watching documentaries, interviews, lectures, debates, and listening to countless testimonials from average people who were having varying degrees of success in their own search for optimal health.

I approached this research with an open mind; ready to change ANYTHING I firmly believed would make me healthier. Many core beliefs I maintained about the food we eat, where it comes from, how it's made and "sold" to us were challenged, and in many cases, changed for the better.

Over the course of this book, I am going to share the biggest discoveries I made along with the most significant adjustments you can make to your current diet that will have POSITIVE health impacts both immediately and for the rest of your life.

One thing you may realize, just as I did – *the solution for optimal health is fairly simple.* Once you understand both the positive and negative consequences associated with eating certain foods, the easier your decisions will be for planning your next meals.

Every single one of us carries DNA that is designed to keep us at a perfect point of health. On a very basic, PRIMAL level, we human beings are "hardwired" to both survive and reproduce, or pass our genetic "blueprints" to future generations so the cycle of life can endure.

Most any creature you see in nature is healthy, perfectly fit, and lean because they INSTINCTIVELY recognize the "fuel" mandatory to their survival and ability to produce offspring. Humans are built the very same way, except for many; we have become DISTRACTED and no longer aware of the foods most suitable for our own survival.

Now is the time to question why we consume poisonous, unhealthy products that only make profits for big corporations at the expense of our health. Let's begin reacquainting ourselves with the foods that have proven VITAL to powering our ancestors through the ages, making it possible for us to be here today.

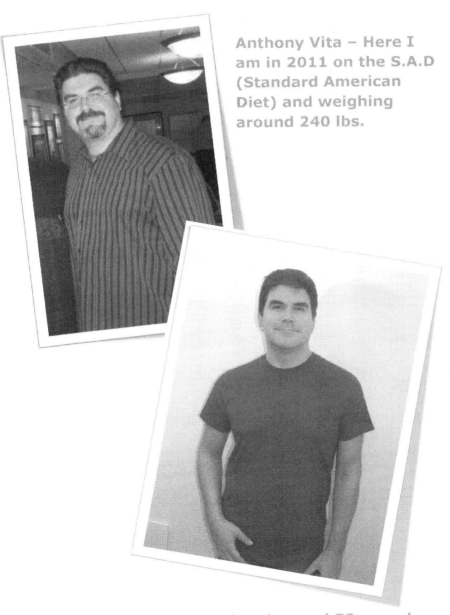

Anthony Vita – Here I am in 2011 on the S.A.D (Standard American Diet) and weighing around 240 lbs.

This is me in 2014 after having dropped 50 pounds and 3 pant sizes. How did I do it? A green smoothie every morning and switching to a mostly plant-based, whole food diet.

ARE YOU HEALTHY?

Now, maybe you're thinking, "I feel fine, I'm healthy". But are you really? See how many of the questions below you can answer "yes"...

- Are you currently taking ANY prescribed pills or medications?
- Do you have acne or any skin conditions?
- Do you suffer from allergies?
- Are you overweight or obese?
- Do you suffer from arthritis, lower back or joint pain?
- Do you frequently experience headaches or migraines?
- Do you get a runny nose, sore throat, cold or sick often?
- Do you have a bowel movement LESS THAN once per day?
- Do you sleep poorly or consistently snore?
- Do you have dark circles under your eyes?
- Do you find yourself "dragging" through each day?

If you can answer "yes" to just ONE of the questions above, it is a clear sign your body is struggling to maintain a healthy balance. For example, if you get sick often, this reveals your immune system has been weakened. If you aren't having at least one bowel movement each day, it's a sign you're not including enough fiber in your diet and, as a result, your body isn't able to cleanse itself efficiently. When your body's defenses and self-cleaning mechanisms are not running optimally, it is much easier for "intruders" to get inside and wreak havoc within your body. Have you ever gotten a virus on your computer?

A computer becomes "infected" once a "barrier" between the computer and the outside world, known as a firewall (or antivirus), fails to intercept an incoming threat. The same happens when our internal "firewall" is not able to protect us from bacterial threats. Keep in mind; contrary to popular belief, *it is not normal for us to get sick on a regular basis.* We'll talk more about this later.

For myself, I could have easily answered "yes" to a few of those questions above for YEARS. I had accepted many of my illnesses as "the new normal" or just part of getting older. However, once I made a few key adjustments to the way I was eating, my health turned around QUICKLY and now I couldn't answer "yes" to even ONE of those questions.

The first adjustment I made was the addition of green smoothies, basically drinking my vegetables on a daily basis. Then, I decided to eliminate all fast food and heavily processed, "junk" foods, such as sodas, snack chips, doughnuts and candy bars. Next, I gradually began centering my meals on plant-based, whole foods, such as potatoes, whole grains, rice, corn and beans. Finally, I took an honest, hard look at the prominent role meat and dairy was playing in my diet and the impacts they were having on my current and, possibly, long-term health.

Over the course of this book I will share the FIVE changes anyone can make to their current diet to SIGNIFICANTLY improve their health, not just for now, but into the future as well.

CHAPTER TWO
Add A Green Smoothie
To Your Day.

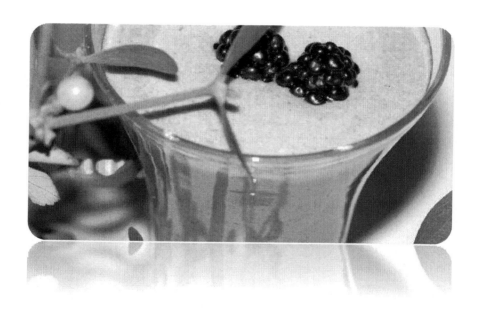

*"When we fail to give our body what it needs,
we create an internal environment that
promotes sickness, disease and obesity."*

THE BENEFITS

- Consume multiple servings of fruits and vegetables at once.

- Help your body to detoxify, get lasting energy and curb cravings.

- Give your body what it needs to fight disease, build new tissues and repair cells.

- Strengthen your immune system, aid digestion and elimination.

Try to think of green smoothies as your internal "bodyguard". When I use that term you may instantly think of celebrities, politicians or any other high profile personality who demands around the clock protection from harm.

Bodyguards are important not only for handling any new threat that may arise but also for DISCOURAGING them from even happening at all. Let's face it; most anyone would think twice before messing with someone who surrounds themselves with bodyguards.

While bodyguards can shield us from physical harm, they unfortunately cannot prevent life-threatening diseases such as colon cancer or heart disease. However, when it comes to healthy foods such as fruits and vegetables, not only can they prevent life threatening disease, they are also proven to FIGHT and REVERSE them as well. Foods do have something in common with personal bodyguards – they both create an "environment" where the undesirable is both handled and prevented.

You see, our body is ALWAYS working to cleanse and heal itself from whatever is causing us to be sick or struggle with disease. Look at what happens when we get a scrape or cut; our skin immediately begins to repair itself – that is all it knows how to do! The same applies to the INSIDE of our bodies as well.

Our body is CONSTANTLY working to correct and compensate for any deficiencies we may have so our health can be restored back to normal levels. The problem is we are not naturally equipping our body with the proper "tools" to repair itself. We continually COMPROMISE our own health because, not only do we fail to give our body what it needs, we further complicate matters by eating foods our body doesn't process efficiently. It would be like trying to mop a wet floor with the sink overflowing; no matter how hard we try, the floor will not get dry.

When we fail to give our body what it needs, we create an internal environment that promotes sickness, disease and obesity. It is important to eat more of the foods that PROMOTE good health and support the many essential systems and chemical reactions occurring at all times inside our body.

If you regularly eat fruits and vegetables, that is fantastic – but are you eating ENOUGH? If you are like me and not fond of eating large amounts of vegetables on a regular basis, adding at least one blended drink loaded with fruits and vegetables each day is an EXCELLENT way to begin your road back to improved health. With just one green smoothie per day you can give your body the kind of tools it needs to create new cells, repair tissues, defend from potential sickness and fight any illnesses you may currently be struggling with.

You may have heard of another popular way to drink vegetables known as "juicing". This is a very different method from making smoothies and it's important to understand the differences, especially for beginners.

BLENDING vs. JUICING

For "juicing" you need a juicer (as opposed to a blender) which basically squeezes the juice out of whatever you add into it. For example, if you feed a stalk of celery to a juicer it will get pulverized so only its juice is extracted, leaving the pulp (or fiber) behind. There is absolutely nothing wrong with this method of extraction; as a matter of fact, juicing can provide you with a much higher concentration of vegetables than blending. However, for beginners, there are some factors to consider.

Juicing has higher startup costs since, in order to juice, you'll need to buy an appliance you don't already own. Also, in order to extract enough juice to fill a single glass you will need to use a great deal of fruits and vegetables, meaning a higher grocery bill. In addition to expense, juicing demands more of your time and attention with food preparation and storage.

For smoothies, all you need is a blender, which you may already own. You don't need large amounts of fruits and vegetables to create a single glass of juice because, unlike juicing, you are blending the WHOLE food instead of just extracting its juice. To make a smoothie, all you do is toss in your fruits and vegetables, nuts or seeds, add some liquid, blend for about a minute and you're ready to start drinking.

Because blending is CHEAPER, FASTER and EASIER, it's not likely to discourage anyone from getting started or stopping once they've begun. With blending a possible concern may be the power of your blender. Low powered blenders (or those with poor blade design) are likely to have a hard time crushing nuts and seeds resulting in grittier, lumpier drinks. So, whether you're shopping for a new blender or looking to buy your first, here are the ones I highly recommend from personal experience.

CHOOSING A BLENDER

In choosing a blender, I would strongly recommend the one that got me started, the NutriBullet. You can find these blenders most anywhere for just under $100 and they are proven to emulsify most anything you throw at it, including nuts and seeds. This blender is also fairly compact, making it easy for travelers to not miss a drink while on the road.

If you've got money to invest in a more versatile blender, I would highly recommend the machine I moved to after the NutriBullet, called the Vitamix. These blenders range anywhere from $350 to $700 depending on the model and go a couple steps beyond making just drinks. The multi-speed functionality and powerful motor make for some very smoothly textured drinks. The Vitamix can also be used to create hot soups and ice cream. I tend to think of the Vitamix as less of a blender and more of a versatile kitchen tool.

SMOOTHIE BASICS

The first thing to remember is that *making smoothies is not an exact science*. Feel free to use any ingredients you like and in any quantity so the drink not only tastes good, but also AGREES with your digestive system as well. Not every drink is for everyone. For example, some may find that combining bananas and broccoli in a smoothie causes gas and bloating. You really won't know how any food combining will affect you until it's tried. As with any food you consume, whether by drinking or eating, *listen to your body.*

If you eat something that doesn't agree with you, simply stop eating it. Right now, I am going to share with you the basic components of a green smoothie and then which ingredients I use so you get an idea of how to get started.

At its most basic level, the drinks I prepare regularly are a blend of *green vegetables*, *fruits*, *nuts, seeds*, *spice* and *raw chocolate*, known as "cacao powder". If you're not a fan of chocolate, you can do without it and just enjoy this as a sweet, banana flavored drink. Cacao powder may be the only ingredient you have to order online as I've found it hard to source locally, especially at a competitive price. It's important to include a variety of ingredients in order to enjoy the many health benefits each generate. Below is a quick chart which outlines the benefits of each ingredient we'll be using:

Spinach

Contains

Beta-carotene, Vitamin C, Vitamin K, Potassium, antioxidants.

Health Benefits

Reduces risk of heart conditions, cataracts, and neurological disorders, anti-inflammatory. Protects against various cancers.

Celery

Contains

Vitamin A, B1, B2, B6 and C, potassium, folic acid, calcium, magnesium, iron, phosphorus, sodium and essential amino acids and oils.

Health Benefits

Equalizes body PH, aids digestion disorders, high blood pressure, arthritis, inflammation, auto-immune disorders, anemia, asthma, skin problems, regulates nervous system, lowers cholesterol, fights cancer, curbs sweet cravings, strong detoxifier.

Cherries

Contains

Beta carotene, vitamin C, boron, antioxidants, melatonin. Potassium.

Health Benefits

Defend against cancer, aids sleep, pain relief, regulates blood sugar, anti-inflammatory.

Banana

Contains

Potassium, tryptophan, serotonin, fiber.

Health Benefits

Lowers high blood pressure, , reduces risk of atherosclerosis and stroke, aids calcium absorption and bone health, fights sleeplessness, mood swings and irritability, helps depression, supports eyesight, aids digestion, prevents constipation.

Dates

Contains

Fiber selenium, manganese, copper, and magnesium iron sulfur, natural sugars.

Health Benefits

Aids digestion, prevents constipation, supports bone health, stimulates growth of friendly bacteria in the intestines, fights anemia and allergies, excellent source of energy, aids nervous system.

Cinnamon

Contains

Antioxidants, calcium, manganese, iron and dietary fiber.

Health Benefits

Reduces cholesterol, blood pressure and blood sugar levels, aids in prevention of dementia (Alzheimer's), relieves arthritis, improves mental alertness, and fights inflammation.

Chia Seeds

Contains

Omega-3, calcium, iron, magnesium, boron, fiber, complete protein source, B Vitamins.

Health Benefits

Aids circulation, heart health, blood sugar and digestion. Chia becomes gelatinous when mixed with liquid and helps bind junk in your intestines for elimination.

Flax Seeds

Contains

Omega-3, magnesium, phosphorus, and copper. Folate, Vitamin B6, lignan phytonutrients.

Health Benefits

Relief of arrhythmia, fights prostate cancer, lowers blood pressure, rheumatoid arthritis, asthma, aids heart health, fights depression and hot flashes

Cacao Powder (raw, organic)

Contains

Antioxidants, theobromine, flavonols.

Health Benefits

Improves blood flow, lowers blood pressure, and reduces risk of heart disease, stroke, and colon cancer. Reduces cell damage and helps prevent Alzheimer's, cancer, improves sugar metabolism, aids chronic fatigue, soothes depression, anxiety and irritability, protects skin against sunburn, boosts cognitive ability, reduces tooth decay, calms coughs and improves vision.

Walnuts

Contains

Vitamin E, vitamin B and magnesium, arginine, fiber.

Health Benefits

Heart health, aids blood flow, boost immune system, lowers bad cholesterol, improves brain function

Optional Ingredients:

Kale

Contains

Fiber, Protein, Antioxidants, Thiamin, Riboflavin, Folate, Iron, Magnesium and Phosphorus, Vitamins A, C, K, B6, Calcium, Potassium, Copper and Manganese.

Health Benefits

Aids in digestion and elimination, helps transporting of oxygen to various parts of the body, cell growth, and liver detoxification, protects against various cancers. Promotes normal bone health, prevents blood clots. Fights Alzheimer's disease, arthritis, asthma and autoimmune disorders, helps lower cholesterol levels, boost immune system, metabolism and hydration, prevents bone loss.

Parsley

Contains

Apigenin, essential oils (Eugenol), folate.

Health Benefits

Antibacterial, reduces cancers, anti-inflammatory, antioxidant, fights allergies, arthritis, liver detoxification, fights bad breath, and reduces blood vessel damage lowering the risk of heart disease

HOW TO MAKE A SMOOTHIE

When shopping for smoothie ingredients, try to buy organic fruits and vegetables when possible. Organic produce are held to higher standards, grown in more nutrient dense soil and should be free from pesticides. Overall, organic foods can be a healthier alternative to conventional produce. However, if you can't source fruits or vegetables organically or can't afford the higher price, don't worry about it. Certainly ANY fruits and vegetables are better than none. Regardless of whether you're buying organic or not, *be sure to thoroughly rinse any produce before chopping and blending to remove pesticides or other residues as much as possible.* Now, let's get started...

Below is a chart showing the ingredients for our smoothie along with serving recommendations based on the type of blender you may be using. Even if you don't have one of the blenders below, chances are yours is similar in size to one of them.

Ingredients	NutriBullet - (Tall cup, 24 oz.)	Vitamix - (48 oz., 6 cups)
Spinach	1 handful	2 handfuls
Celery	1 stalk chopped	2 stalks chopped
Cherries	4 (frozen)	6 (frozen)
Banana	1 frozen	2 frozen
Dates	3	6
Cinnamon	2-3 dashes	2-3 dashes
Chia Seeds	1 tbsp.	1 tbsp.
Flax Seeds	1 tbsp.	1 tbsp.
Walnuts	1 small handful	1 small handful
Cacao Powder	1 tbsp.	1 tbsp.
Spring Water	Fill to Max Line	Fill to top, or as needed.

Next, I will take you through each step of creating this drink and then share ways you can modify it to both maximize nutrition and taste:

Step 1: Add Greens: First, let's add in the green vegetables. I try to include a couple varieties of greens in each drink to maximize nutritional benefits. You can use only one green if that works best for you and your budget or no greens at all if you feel like you eat enough throughout the day already. For this drink you'll need *spinach* and *celery*. Since greens can occupy the bulk of your blender space, you will need to determine how much to use. If you have a smaller blender, you can refer to amounts recommended for the NutriBullet. If your blender is larger you can use the amounts recommended for the Vitamix. The first thing to do is literally grab a handful or two of spinach and toss into the blender. Next up, chop one to two celery stalks and add as well. If at least half of your blender is filled with greens, you're doing fine.

Step 2: Add Fruits: Since I prefer chilled drinks, certain fruits are frozen ahead of time. For example, I'll buy *bananas*, wait for them to get spotted brown, peel then freeze in an air tight container or freezer bag. Even if you're not freezing bananas, it's very important to let them get spotted brown as this makes them sweeter, and helps mask the taste of the greens. For *cherries*, I always buy them frozen and include around 4-6. Next, add 3-6 dates. Organic dates may be hard to find, however, any variety of conventional pitted dates will work just as well. Feel free to add as many dates as you can fit or afford. The more you add, the sweeter your drink will be.

Step 3: Add Dry Ingredients: Now it's time for the Chia and Flax seeds, as well as nuts/seeds, cacao powder and cinnamon. If you don't already have them, be sure to pick up a set of measuring cups with teaspoons/tablespoons so you can add in dry ingredients with more consistency. For flax seeds, be sure to buy them already ground (milled); otherwise you will need to grind them ahead of time in a coffee grinder or blender. Also, be sure to store your flax seeds in a cool place, such as the refrigerator or

freezer. Chia seeds do not require any special storage and are used "as is" in seed form. For this drink, add 1 tbsp. each to the blender, and then add 2-3 dashes of cinnamon to taste. Next, add in a small handful of walnuts. If you don't have these, any nut will do particularly almonds, Brazil nuts or pecans. Although the recommended serving size of cacao powder is 2 ½ tbsps., I've found that using just 1 tbsp. is plenty to give your drink a rich, chocolate taste. Keep in mind that chocolate is a stimulant, so I wouldn't recommend adding cacao to any drinks close to bedtime.

Step 4: Add Liquids: I usually add the liquids last; in this case, try to use the freshest water you can find (100% natural spring water is best). Initially I bought spring water by the gallon and then invested in a water filtration system so I could use the water coming out of the tap instead of having to purchase it on a regular basis. If you're using the Nutribullet, be mindful of the "max line" and do not exceed or you will create quite a mess. With the Vitamix, I typically add water until it's all the way to the top, or six cups. The more water you add, the more smooth the drink will be. The less liquid, the more dense and thick it will be.

Step 5: Blend: If you're using a Nutribullet, blend this mixture for about 20 seconds to a minute. In the Vitamix, I usually start it off on the highest setting for about 30 seconds, and then turn it down to about 6-7 and wait until the "snapping" of the dates, nuts or celery subsides, usually another 30 seconds. Try not to blend the drink for more than a minute as the continued friction may result in a warmer drink. The end result should be a delicious, chocolate-banana smoothie that your body will thank you for!

After you take a few sips and get a feel for the flavors you may want to improve it. Below are ideas for how you can customize any drink to your liking:

CUSTOMIZE YOUR SMOOTHIE

Not Sweet Enough? Add more dates, bananas or organic cane sugar.

Not Cold Enough? Add ice, cold water or frozen fruits.

Too Green? Add more fruit or cacao powder for a deeper, chocolate taste.

Too Watery? Use less water, blend for a shorter amount of time or at lower power, add more chia seeds or nut milk.

Too thick? Blend for longer; add more water or include fewer bananas or milk.

Rotate Greens, Add Variety: Try switching up the contents of your drink from time to time. This will not only prevent tiring of the same drink every day but will also help you reap the many benefits that other fruits and vegetables have to offer. As you can see from the chart earlier which detailed all the ingredients, each plant carries its own health benefits (vitamins, minerals, phytonutrients) so it's important to have VARIETY so that you can enjoy as many benefits as possible. For example, maybe one week you use the greens listed in this book. Perhaps in a couple of weeks swap the *celery* for *parsley*. Then maybe another week you can swap the *spinach* with *collard greens, broccoli or kale*. Feel free to experiment and try new drinks and, as always, listen to your body in case something doesn't taste good or agree with you.

Determine your "base": No matter what kind of smoothie you make, it's important to include fruits with "soluble fiber", to make your smoothie creamier. This is what's referred to as the "base" of your drink because it helps bridge the gap between the often bitter greens and sweet fruits. Recommended fruits are bananas, mangos, blueberries, strawberries, peaches, pears, or melons. If you don't like adding sweet fruit to your smoothie, you can always add a slice of avocado, which also provides a creamy texture.

Quick Shopping List for "The Vital Blend" Smoothie:

Veg.	Fruits:	Spice:	Super foods:	Nuts:	Liquid:
Spinach	Bananas	Cinnamon	Chia Seeds	Walnuts	Spring Water
Celery	Cherries (frozen)		Flax Seeds (ground)		Filtered Water
	Dates		Cacao Powder (raw, organic)		

Just remember…

- Try to buy organic whenever possible, however, any produce is better than none. Organic is <u>not</u> a requirement.

- Always thoroughly wash any produce to reduce consumption of pesticides or other residues.

- Allow bananas to get spotted brown. Freeze for chilled drinks.

- Cacao may be hard to find locally but great deals are online.

- With dates, make sure they're pitted before blending.

- Try to buy ground flax seeds; otherwise you'll need to blend ahead.

- Store flax seeds in the refrigerator or freezer to maintain freshness.

SECTION HIGHLIGHTS (Ch. 2)

- Today, the foods we eat are mostly PRODUCTS made and sold by CORPORATIONS. Like any other product a corporation sells, they are driven by certain principles to be successful; manufacture their products as cheaply as possible, convince customers they need it and then advertise it to them ENDLESSLY.

- Our body is DESIGNED to heal itself, both inside and out.

- When we fail to give our body what it needs to heal itself we increase our risk of developing illnesses and disease.

- The vitamins and nutrients found in fruits and vegetables both FIGHT & REVERSE common illness and disease.

- Green smoothies are like an internal "bodyguard" protecting our health from harmful, foreign invaders.

- Because blending is CHEAPER, FASTER and EASIER, it's not likely to discourage anyone from getting started or stopping once they've begun.

- Organic produce are held to higher standards, grown in more nutrient dense soil and without the use of pesticides. While buying organic fruits and vegetables for smoothies is optimal, ANY fruits and vegetables are better than none.

- Smoothie making is not an exact science. Mix fruits and vegetables that not only taste good but agree with your digestion.

- LISTEN to your body and remove any foods that don't make you feel well, regardless if you're eating or drinking them.

CHAPTER THREE
Eat Mostly Plant-Based Foods

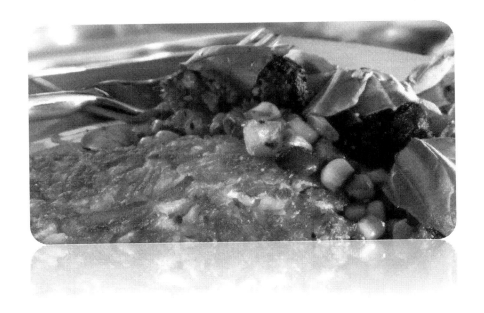

"When we consume natural, whole foods our stomach is filled, our hunger disappears, our body is SATISFIED, we're properly nourished and don't overeat. In other words, NO COUNTING CALORIES..."

Every time we eat there are risks involved, much like when we drive. As soon as we climb into a car our risk of physical harm increases. Depending on how, when and where we drive the risks escalate further. Speeding down the interstate during rush hour in icy weather poses more risks than driving around the corner on a sunny day.

When it comes to foods that are nutritious, safe and REDUCE our risk of sickness and disease, there is nothing better than plant-based, WHOLE foods. Whole foods originate from the GROUND and do not include any added chemicals, artificial flavors, or other harmful ingredients.

Below are examples of plant-based, whole foods:

Fruits	Berries, apples, oranges, pears, melons, grapes, bananas, figs, mangoes, peaches, pineapples, raisins, dates.
Vegetables	Tomatoes, spinach, kale, celery, carrots, broccoli, artichokes, peppers, squash, lettuce, Brussels sprouts, cabbage, onions, cauliflower.
Starches	Potatoes (white or sweet)
Grains	Rice, oats, barley, wheat, buckwheat, millet, corn, pasta, quinoa (a seed).
Legumes	Beans, peas, lentils

Plant-based, whole foods do not increase the likelihood of disease by promoting an environment inside of our body that encourages cancer cell growth, clogged arteries, obesity or constipation. Why would you not want to eat these foods or, at least, eat MORE of them than the foods that increase health risks?

WHY WE EAT

When we start feeling hungry our body is telling us; "*We need more energy*". It is important to understand which foods provide optimal "fuel" for our body so we can make better decisions on how to properly nourish it.

It's so easy to get distracted and not know where to start in eating healthy. Everywhere you turn people are talking about various diets, counting calories, getting enough protein, going gluten free, or eating like a caveman. It's very easy to be overwhelmed by all this information and ultimately decide to do NOTHING and continue our bad habits. So, how can we eat and be sure we're getting the proper amount of calories, fiber, nutrients and protein?

One of the most basic things you need to know is WE EAT FOR ENERGY. *When we consume the most optimal foods for energy, all of the proteins, vitamins, minerals and fiber required to maintain proper health are naturally built-in as well.* There's an old phrase, "kill two birds with one stone".

This happens when we accomplish two actions by only setting out to do one. For example, let's say you make an effort to walk a mile every day and on that walk you picked up some food at the grocery store. Not only did you exercise, but you were able to go food shopping as well. In terms of eating, when you choose optimal sources of energy food, your body is also nourished with all the required vitamins, minerals, protein and fiber to maintain proper health.

When we consume natural, whole foods our stomach is filled, our hunger disappears, our body is SATISFIED, we're properly nourished and don't overeat. In other words, NO COUNTING CALORIES or having to worry about what diet we should be on. When we start eating correctly, our body makes adjustments, our cravings disappear and we rebound, just like a withered flower as soon as it receives fresh water.

THE HEALTHY FOOD "SYMPHONY"

When we eat a whole food, such as an apple or stalk of celery, our body knows EXACTLY how to sort out all the nutrients and vitamins it contains. Like a symphony, all the individual parts work together in HARMONY, namely proteins, vitamins, minerals, phytonutrients, carbohydrates, sugars, fats and fiber.

Consuming WHOLE foods allows our bodies to function at optimum levels because it is able to make use of all these various nutrients to build and repair cells, flush toxins and supply us with energy at the same time. Eating plant-based, whole foods is a win-win for our body. We get the energy needed to work or play and our body gets what it needs to make certain we remain healthy and our defenses are strong.

Let's take a closer look at the "players" in this whole food symphony to better understand how they help us:

PROTEIN

Our body uses protein to build new tissues, repair damaged cells and a host of many other essential functions. *Proteins found in plant-based foods are, by far, the best suited for human health.* We can look to nature for confirmation on this as plants are so nutrient dense they EASILY meet the protein needs of our planet's largest animals including giraffes, cows, elephants and hippopotamuses. There is no reason to believe the protein needs of humans can't be satisfied by plants as well.

In the first two years of a human's life, when we're at our GREATEST need for protein and actually DOUBLING in size, we depend on human breast milk which is only 5% protein. As we grow and consume foods like rice (8% protein), oatmeal (15% protein) or beans (27% protein) you can see how EASILY our protein requirements are met to maintain proper growth, health and nutrition. This is the reason why any cases of protein deficiency among humans are virtually UNKNOWN in recorded history.

Sadly, the amount of protein we're told that we need has been greatly EXAGGERATED and fallen victim to the marketing tactics of, you guessed it, greedy CORPORATIONS looking to make a profit and sell more products.

You see, unlike fat, our body does not store protein. Once we consume more protein than our body needs it gets passed through our liver and kidneys and into the toilet. Not only does this overwork our liver and potentially lead to problems such as kidney stones or osteoporosis, it also makes for pretty expensive urine, particularly with the regular consumption of supplements such as protein powders.

The bottom line is, when we intake more of ANYTHING than our body can handle efficiently, the excess amount is treated like a POISON. I know it's hard to think of protein as potentially "toxic" because we're accustomed to hearing it's among the ONLY things we need to be concerned about. The truth is there is no single, isolated nutrient we need to stay focused on. *Always remember it is a "symphony" or BLEND of nutrients that work to our benefit.*

VITAMINS and MINERALS

An entire book can be written about the importance of vitamins and minerals to our health and well-being. Acting together, they have literally HUNDREDS of roles within our body. They help create strong bones, heal wounds, and boost our immune system. They also convert food into energy, and repair cellular damage.

If you made an effort to learn what each vitamin and mineral does for our body it would be overwhelming and confusing. To keep things simple, as with protein, you don't need to be concerned about any one, isolated vitamin or mineral. Just know they all work in HARMONY and it's important to eat as many plant-based foods as possible to reap their numerous benefits.

FATS

As with protein, plant-based foods contain the healthiest fats for human consumption, known as polyunsaturated fats (Omega-3 and Omega-6). These fats are considered "essential" because we can't make them ourselves so we depend on our food to acquire them. These fats help our cell membranes to remain strong and healthy; without them, we increase our risk of a compromised immune system or developing heart disease, obesity, even cancer.

The safest and healthiest way to consume these essential fats is by eating plant-based foods where they are found in the correct amounts and surrounded by vitamins, minerals, fibers, antioxidants, and other phytochemicals to make them a balanced nutritional option.

The downside to fat is when we consume the type that work AGAINST us. Saturated fat is highest in animal-derived foods or refined vegetable oils such as meat, milk, butter, cheese and olive oil. Upon eating these fats they are absorbed by the intestine into our bloodstream and then transported to the millions of cells intended for storing body fat. The conversion happens so effortlessly, if you were to analyze a sample of someone's body fat tissue you could easily identify the kind of fats they typically consume. For example, with someone who eats margarine you can detect what's known as "trans" fats in their fatty tissues. You could also take a blood sample from someone who's just eaten a cheeseburger with fries and literally see the fat in the vial holding their blood.

It is this type of fat that makes our blood become more vicious, or thick, and can eventually lead to high blood pressure, obesity and heart disease.

SUGAR

You will hear many claims that sugar is bad for us. However, *sugar (glucose) is ESSENTIAL to every single cell in our body, which uses it for fuel.* There are two important things to keep in mind about sugar.

First, sugar is an ISOLATED nutrient. For example, apples have sugar but they also have fiber, vitamin C and calcium, among other things. When we eat an apple our body is enjoying that "symphony" of nutrients I talked about earlier. This is the BEST way to consume sugar, when it's contained within a natural, whole food. One major reason for this is due to fiber. Have you ever eaten something containing a lot of sugar and then felt really tired afterwards? This is because you consumed a large amount of isolated sugar, delivered directly into your bloodstream, supplying you with loads of energy (called a "sugar high") and when it ran out, you "crashed".

When you consume sugar WITH fiber, it's like jumping out of an airplane with a parachute. The fiber acts as a "time-release", so the sugar EASES its way into your bloodstream giving you SUSTAINED energy, preventing a "crash".

The second thing to remember about sugar is that we feel extreme satisfaction when consuming it because our taste buds are DESIGNED to detect and enjoy sugar (carbohydrates). Why do you think CORPORATIONS spend millions of dollars finding the right combination of sugar, salt and fat to addict us to their potato chips and soft drinks? They know the science too.

Most of the problems with sugar are the "company" it keeps with other ingredients. Sugar is like the good kid who hangs out with the troublemakers. Have you ever known a good, honest person who gets wrapped up with the wrong crowd and winds up getting in trouble themselves? It's very similar to what happens with us and sugar. Because we derive so much pleasure from sugar, we seek it out but not always in the best manner. When we eat an orange we get the sugar, along with fiber, calcium and other vitamins. When we eat jellybeans we get the sugar, along with artificial flavoring and other CHEMICALS. Because jellybeans don't fill our stomach or meet our nutrient needs (like oranges would), our hunger drive remains unsatisfied and we tend to eat MORE of the jellybeans and the "junk" associated with them.

While sugar is not the "bad guy" it's been made out to be, it is not a health food either. Always be aware of the "context" in which you're eating sugary foods and try to consume most of your sugar from plant-based sources. Adding some table sugar to your oatmeal or marinara sauce is not a problem. Wouldn't nature have played a cruel joke on humans if our cells needed sugar for fuel and our tongues were designed to taste it, yet we couldn't have any?

CARBOHYDRATES

"Carbs" or "starches", such as potatoes and rice, are sugar too, except they are known as "complex" sugars. On a molecular level carbohydrates consist of longer sugar "chains" than those simpler ones found in fruits. Think of it like a train – ever been stuck at a railroad crossing and had to wait for the train to go by before you could cross the track?

This is very similar to how carbs and sugar work as fuel inside our body. The more cars on a train, the longer we wait for it to pass. The more sugar "chains" we consume, the more sustained our energy and longer we can go before feeling tired again. Ever waited for a train that was only a couple of cars long? You didn't have to wait very long for it to pass, did you? This is what happens when you eat simple sugars, such as those found in fruit. A single apple will satisfy you, but only for a short period of time.

This explains why eating complex carbs (starches), such as sweet potatoes, are more satisfying and provide more lasting energy than a single fruit. It's because of the amount of carbohydrates, or fuel, it contains.

You will hear some claim that "carbs make you fat". This is simply not true because, if it were, history would clearly show massive obesity in the billions of traditional Asian populations who have lived off rice based meals for thousands of years. When consuming carbohydrates, our body digests them into simple sugars which are then delivered to the trillions of cells in our body for energy purposes. Any carbs consumed in excess of our needs are generally burned off as heat through day-to-day physical movements. Humans are not very efficient at converting sugar into fat, like cows or pigs. This is why they tend to grow very rapidly and, not surprisingly, we find them ideal "food animals". However, *just know that plant-based carbs = energy and satisfaction*. Plant-based foods with the most carbohydrates are beans, legumes, sweet potatoes, corn, rice, barley and oats.

FIBER

Fiber is known as "nature's broom" because it helps move our bowels and keeps waste (toxins) moving through our intestines so it can eventually be eliminated. When we don't eat enough fiber our waste can't exit quick enough and it starts to fester inside our body, often leading to infections and a variety of other health issues. The longer waste sits in our intestines waiting for a "broom" to push it along; the more time toxins and bacteria have to form and work their way back into our system.

What would happen if you didn't take out the garbage regularly? No doubt it would begin piling up, overflowing, stinking and perhaps attracting flies or worse. The same happens inside our bodies.

Virtually all diseases are triggered by toxins entering the bloodstream through our intestinal lining. As a result, our liver gets overworked attempting to remove these toxins, our blood experiences "toxemia" and this is spread to tissues throughout our body resulting in everything from mood disorders, skin blemishes, and bad breath to much more serious, life-threatening illnesses and diseases.

The toxins in our body come from a variety of places including the food we eat, the water we drink and even the air we breathe. This is why maintaining a healthy colon is ESSENTIAL to our overall well-being. Our colon is more than just an organ that eliminates waste; it is a KEY part of our digestive process. Once our colon begins working less than optimally, our digestion becomes disrupted and the essential vitamins, minerals, and other nutrients our body depends on to grow and thrive are no longer absorbed properly.

When we don't eat enough fiber, we find ourselves straining to move our bowels, leading to a host of even more health issues including hemorrhoids, varicose veins or diverticulitis. Problems such as these are common in America but have been virtually UNKNOWN in Africa or Asia, why? In those countries, meals are centered on plant-based foods such as rice and corn, which are ABUNDANT in fiber and keep their bodies routinely cleansed.

Fiber is only found in plant foods and provides yet another tremendous benefit, apart from bowel cleansing. Fiber helps grow the GOOD BACTERIA already living in our gut. Having our good bacteria outnumber the bad kind helps to promote and maintain optimal health.

SECTION HIGHLIGHTS (Ch.3)

- When it comes to foods that are nutritious, safe and REDUCE our risk of sickness and disease, there is nothing better than plant-based, WHOLE foods.

- Whole foods are fruits, vegetables, starches, grains, and legumes.

- We eat for energy. When we consume the most optimal foods for energy, all of the proteins, vitamins, minerals and fiber required to maintain proper health are naturally built-in as well.

- Proteins, vitamins and minerals, carbohydrates, sugar and fiber work together in harmony, like a "symphony", inside our body.

- Plant based protein is the best source of protein for humans.

- Our body does not store protein and any excess amounts are treated as toxins and flushed from our body.

- Plant-based fats are the best source of fat for humans.

- Every cell in our body uses sugar as fuel.

- Sugar is best when consumed as part of a whole food, such as fruit, where it's surrounded by other nutrients such as fiber, vitamins and minerals.

- Carbohydrates, such as rice and potatoes, are "complex" sugars and provide us with lasting energy and satisfaction between meals.

- Virtually all diseases are triggered by toxins entering the bloodstream through our intestinal lining.

- The consumption of fiber, or "nature's broom", is the best way to ensure our colon and intestines are cleaned regularly. When we don't eat enough of the foods that promote an optimal diet, we become nutritionally imbalanced and more susceptible to symptoms of disease.

CHAPTER FOUR
Stop Eating "Junk" Foods

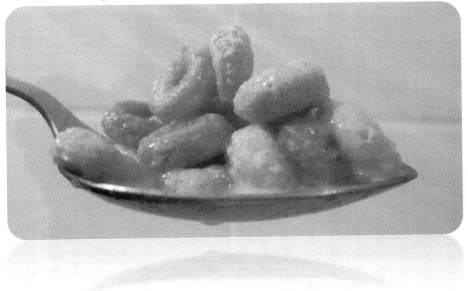

"Not only do these foods taste good, they contain CHEMICALS and are designed to ADDICT us."

THE JUNK LIST

Fast Food, Fried Foods, Microwave Meals, Chocolate Bars, Candy, Packaged Chips, Cakes, Pies, Cookies, Ice Cream, Doughnuts, Sodas, Fruit punch, Milkshakes and the like.

So what makes a food "junk"? Quite simply, a food is considered "junk" when it offers little to no nutritional benefits. When we eat these foods, our body receives little nourishment – meaning we don't give ourselves much to help grow, repair or replenish blood cells or skin tissues. We certainly aren't doing anything to strengthen our immune system, prevent or even fight diseases. And quite often junk foods make us constipated and unable to keep our intestines clean due to their lack of fiber. When consumed in excess, these foods can lead to all sorts of health problems from acne to obesity and from heart disease to cancer.

If these foods didn't taste so good, it would be easy to stay away from them. However, THAT is the problem. Not only do these foods taste good, they contain CHEMICALS and are designed to ADDICT us.

Take blueberry muffins, for example. While working my hectic corporate job, I looked forward to having a blueberry muffin on most mornings. I LOVE blueberries so, of course, having them in a muffin along with coffee was my favorite way to start the day (and usually the only thing I ate until lunch).

But think about it, if food companies had to use REAL blueberries in their muffins it would cost them a FORTUNE. Plus, how would they prevent all those berries from quickly spoiling? Well, the solution is quite simple, don't use REAL blueberries!

Instead of using actual fruit, a blueberry "flavor" is created in a laboratory. To substitute for the missing, natural ingredients they rely on chemicals, commonly found in non-food products, to get the job done. When it comes to blueberry muffins, it's common to see ingredients such as "Red #40", "Blue #1" and "Blue #2" or worse, "Propylene Glycol" to give the "blueberry illusion". By the way, outside of the food industry, the latter is the same chemical used to winterize RVs! (recreational vehicles)

You see, food corporations and fast food giants have realized that by targeting our most PRIMAL taste desires they can get us to eat just about ANYTHING. By working their lab "magic", food scientists have found ways to include such things as silly putty and wood pulp in our food and make it taste AMAZING by a clever combination of the three pillars on which these companies survive – SALT, SUGAR and FAT.

Food scientists spend MILLIONS of dollars and many hours in laboratories testing for what's known as the "bliss point" with sugar, the "mouth feel" for fat or the "flavor burst" for salt.

Here are some shocking facts on how chemicals are used in everyday foods:

- **(Partially) Hydrogenated Vegetable Oils** – This is among the WORST ingredients you will EVER find on a food label due to the "trans fats" associated with it. This all happens when regular vegetable oil (fat) goes through a process called "hydrogenation". In this process, hydrogen is mixed with vegetable oil turning it solid at room temperature. In terms of food production, this helps maintain not only texture but a longer shelf life and can be found in everything from fast foods to crackers, frozen pizzas and microwave popcorn. Just as the oil has become more solid, so does our BLOOD when this type of chemical enters the bloodstream, raising "bad" cholesterol levels and increasing our risk of a stroke or heart attack. To put it bluntly, hydrogenated oils are closer to a PLASTIC than to any real food. Maybe this is why the FDA has deemed trans-fats not "generally recognized as safe" for use in food at ANY level.

- **MSG (Monosodium Glutamate)** is commonly used as a flavor-enhancer in MANY common grocery store items from instant soups to snack chips and used HEAVILY at fast food restaurants. MSG is typically used to fatten lab rats for testing purposes and, no doubt, it has the same effect on humans. In addition, MSG is linked to asthma, hives, skin rashes, vomiting, heart irregularities and even seizures.

- **BHT/BHA (Butylated Hydroxytoluene/Butylated Hydroxyanisole)** is used in embalming fluid and as fuel in jets. BHA is toxic to our organs and linked to cancer. Where is it commonly found? Pepperoni in fast food pizzas, among other places.

- **Sodium Nitrites** are often used to preserve meats such as pepperoni, ham, bacon and sausage toppings. Such additives have been linked to cancer in humans and recently declared a Group 1 carcinogen by the World Health Organization (same category as tobacco).

- **BPA (Bisphenol A)** is something you will not find listed on any ingredient label, because it "leaches" from the plastic bottles and cans of various products used and sold in some restaurants and grocery stores. For example, plastic water bottles or tomato sauce cans used by many fast food pizza chains could have BPA, a substance that increases your risk for cardiovascular disease, breast cancer, prostate cancer, diabetes and a slew of other medical problems.

- **Diacetyl (DA)** is an ingredient used to create the buttery aroma and flavor in microwave popcorn, margarine, candy, baked goods, and even pet food. DA easily penetrates the precious "blood-brain" barrier, a layer of cells that is supposed to keep harmful substances from entering the brain but allows other helpful materials to cross. DA is linked to nerve damage and also a condition known as "Popcorn Lung".

- **Aspartame** is the classic example of an FDA approved ingredient that's common to thousands of products yet one of the biggest DANGERS to human health. Marketed as a weight loss aid, aspartame is an artificial sweetener (known as NutraSweet or Equal) and common to most diet sodas. One startling fact is how aspartame can turn to formaldehyde upon entering the body. Well no wonder the reported side-affects read like a who's who of serious health problems, ranging from breast cancer to multiple sclerosis. If you need to sweeten that drink or meal, don't be afraid to add natural sweeteners such as honey, agave, stevia or just plain table sugar.

- **Cellulose** is an ingredient you will find in many pre-packaged foods and is listed as "added fiber" on ingredient labels. Earlier I mentioned how plant-based foods have fiber that aids our digestion. However, as with the blueberry example earlier, food companies stand to lose profits if fiber from REAL food was used. You know what also has fiber? Trees! Yes, "wood pulp" is much cheaper to source and doesn't spoil as quickly as the fiber from real, plant-based foods. The bad news is that wood pulp offers ZERO nutritional benefits and is indigestible by the human body, leaving us hungry for more. On the contrary, REAL fiber from plant-based foods produces "acetate" in our colon, which messages feelings of satiety (feeling "full") to our brain, supporting appetite suppression.

- **Dimethylpolysiloxane**, or "silly putty", is commonly found in soft drinks and MANY fast foods as well as silicone caulks, adhesives, and aquarium sealants, heat transfer fluids, polishes, cosmetics, and hair conditioners. Since it was legally approved in 1998 there have been no tests conducted on its impact on human health.

- **4-methylimidazole, or 4-Mel**, is not something you will see listed on soda labels; however, it does appear under the guise of "caramel coloring." Studies have shown this chemical can lead to cancer. While the FDA has set no legal limit for the use of 4-Mel in products, the state of California has imposed cancer warning labels for any products sold within the state exposing customers to more than 29 micrograms per day. Consumer Reports already found sodas using this ingredient, with some exceeding "safe" levels and without warnings on the label.

Can you see how eating foods made in a laboratory come with their share of health risks? Why shouldn't this be surprising when you consider the amount of CHEMICALS used in processed, junk foods these days? Maybe now you can better understand why I claimed we are all being literally POISONED at the start of this book.

Even though these chemicals are being used at levels approved "safe" by the Food & Drug Administration (FDA), who eats just ONE serving or ONE food at a time? How common is it to eat a fast food sandwich along with chips and a soda? How safe are those isolated levels when consumed in COMBINATION? And how safe is it when this type of food is eaten regularly or even a few times a week or a month? The answer is - nobody knows for sure because testing has never been conducted at this level. Actually, the only testing being performed on the consumption of chemical foods is on you and me whenever we eat them!

Since junk foods don't provide much nourishment or fill our stomachs like real food, we remain HUNGRY. This is why we tend to OVER EAT these types of foods. In addition to the many illnesses and diseases we place ourselves at risk for; the overconsumption of these foods leads to weight gain due to excessive CALORIES.

EMPTY CALORIES

You've probably heard the term "empty calories", but what does it mean exactly and how does it relate to weight gain?

Basically, we gain weight by consuming more calories than our body is able to burn off. The problem overweight or obese people have is they are consuming WAY more calories than they realize and so the weight stays on regardless of how much strenuous exercise they do. It's like trying to empty a swimming pool with a coffee cup at one end while a garden hose pumps in more water at the other.

Before we get too far, let's define a "calorie". Basically, a calorie is a unit of measurement. In the case of food, a calorie is a unit of ENERGY. For example, just like your car may get 15 miles for every gallon of gas, a teaspoon of sugar would be equal to 15 units of energy, or calories. *Everything we eat is measured in calories because, as I mentioned earlier, we eat for ENERGY.*

As a general rule, know that one gram of carbohydrate has 4 calories and a gram of fat has 9 calories. This means when you eat foods high in fat you are effortlessly more than DOUBLING your caloric intake.

One of the most popular foods on the planet is the potato. Unfortunately, most people prefer consuming them fried in fatty oils, such as with fries or potato chips. What does this mean in terms of calories?

In the chart on the next page you can see how eating one medium potato is 153 calories. To reach the same amount of calories eating potato chips, we only need to eat about 12-15 chips. Who eats just a few potato chips? I know for myself and others it's so easy to BINGE on chips and eat half a bag at one time!

When it comes to your average fries, you can see below how eating almost HALF as much fried potato gives you more than DOUBLE the amount of calories. When we start comparing calories from fries with the most popular fast-food chain on the planet, McDonalds, it gets even more shocking. Consuming one large order of McDonald's fries is the caloric equivalent of eating nearly 3½ medium potatoes!

Food	Weight	Calories
Medium Potato	213 g (7.5 oz.)	153
Potato Chips (12-15)	28.4 g (1 oz.)	152
Average Fries	117 g (4.12 oz.)	365
*McDonalds Small Fries	71 g (2.5 oz.)	230 .
*McDonalds Large Fries	154 g (5.4 oz.)	500

* McDonald's USA Nutrition Facts for Popular Menu Items.

I know what you're probably thinking, "McDonald's fries taste SO good! Eating a regular potato isn't the same thing!" Believe me, I get it. I think McDonalds fries are the best in the world too. However, I'm trying to get across how EASY it is to over consume CALORIES with just a small amount of food.

But it gets worse.

Because we're not eating food with much DENSITY our stomach doesn't fill up. This means we keep eating until our body is satisfied and "signals" it's time to stop.

You see, our stomachs have nutrient and stretch "sensors" which signal us once we've eaten enough food to physically fill our stomach and reach our nutrient requirements. Once this happens we feel "full" and don't feel comfortable eating anything until our stomach empties again.

The problem with eating refined foods like potato chips is they are high in calories, lacking in nutrients and low in DENSITY, meaning they don't physically fill our stomach so we feel like eating MORE. The more we eat the more calories we consume.

As an example, let's say the chart below represents what two people, Joe and Victoria, eat for lunch on any given day:

Joe's Lunch	TOTAL CALORIES
2 medium baked potatoes (15 oz.) Calories = 306 Salad, w/vegetables (7.3 oz.) Calories = 40 Spring Water (12 oz.) Calories = 0	**346 Calories from 34 oz.**
Victoria's Lunch	
Large McDonalds Fries (5.4 oz) Calories = 500 McDonalds Big Mac (7.6 oz) Calories = 550 Coke (12oz. can) Calories = 143	**1193 calories from 25 oz.**

Right away you can see Joe is consuming FAR fewer calories than Victoria but is eating MORE food, meaning he is likely to feel more satisfied and eat less over the course of the day. Victoria is likely to feel hungrier sooner and wind up eating more than Joe. By the end of the day Victoria could easily consume TEN times more calories than Joe, but actually consume LESS food. If this pattern of eating continues day after day, perhaps for months or even years on end, these excess calories will result in weight GAIN.

Here is another scenario where Joe and Victoria eat the SAME amount of food, yet one still manages to consume more calories. Let's say they both eat a bowl of pasta (180 calories), however, Victoria adds two tablespoons of olive oil to hers. Because olive oil is mostly saturated fat and twice the amount of calories per gram than the pasta, Victoria is now consuming 240 MORE calories than Joe. In order for Joe to consume another 240 calories he would have to eat over two pounds of lettuce or 2 more potatoes. Since Joe's stomach is already full from the single bowl of pasta, he's not likely to eat that much additional food.

Now you may be thinking, "Victoria has always been pretty thin, she won't get fat." This may be true to some extent. Some people have what's known as "skinny genes", where their genetics simply don't "allow" them to add weight easily. This type of person is more likely to gain a pound or two per year, so that over a 20 year period they've gained 20 pounds. For people with "hefty genes", they are more likely to add those same 20 pounds in only two or three years.

If you want to lose weight or keep the pounds off, it's important to maximize the calories you consume so they physically fill your stomach, while supplying nourishment and energy at the same time. The more you consume of foods that fail to deliver what your body needs, the more you promote that internal environment, mentioned earlier, where you become out of balance and set the stage for weight gain.

Foods such as olive oil or fries are considered "rich" because they are HIGHLY concentrated with fat. These are also highly processed, or refined, foods because they've been stripped of their primary nutrients. To make olive oil, over a thousand olives are basically squeezed so only their oil is saved, leaving behind all other nutrients, including fiber, vitamins and minerals. If you had just eaten olives, the fiber in them would have helped fill your stomach, unlike only the oil from those olives, which slips in practically undetected, easily adding more calories.

This scenario plays out time and time again and is the reason why most Americans struggle with their weight. It's not because their body is malfunctioning, they have mental problems or bad genes. It's because they don't realize how many calories they're consuming at each meal.

As you can see in the chart on the next page, once the line from eating plant-based, whole foods to meat, dairy and highly refined/processed foods is crossed, the caloric density increases while the food density decreases. Unfortunately, it is the calorie dense foods we tend to CENTER most of our meals around and one of the primary reasons why we face critical health issues today.

If you are really serious about losing weight or reversing any kind of illness or disease, it begins with recognizing where your current diet falls in the chart below. If most of what you eat is below the black line, your risk of becoming obese or developing heart disease is greatly increased than if most of your meals (and calories) are derived from foods above the line.

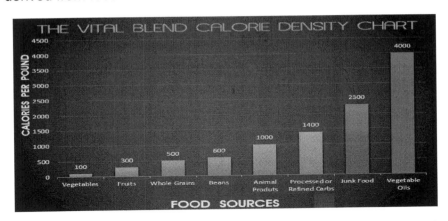

Food Group	Calories Per Pound
Vegetables	100
Fruits	300
Whole Grains	500
Beans	600
Animal Products	1000
Processed/Refined Carbs	1400
Junk Food	2300
Vegetable Oils	4000

If your diet is centered on the foods below the black line, what types of adjustments can you make in order to move above the line? Start by swapping out one high calorie food for a low calorie one. You don't have to change EVERYTHING you're eating at once, begin one food or meal at a time.

For example, if you start each day with a bacon, egg and cheese biscuit, try having a bowl of oatmeal instead, topped with your favorite fruit along with a spoonful of honey and dash or two of cinnamon. The fast food biscuit is close to 500 calories and your oatmeal will approach 200 calories. Right away you've shaved 300 calories off your day and are that much closer to seeing positive results.

For some it may be swapping out cans of soda with spring water. With each soda containing around 150 calories, you could save a CONSIDERABLE amount of calories each day just by stopping that one habit. By going this route you will accomplish the following:

1) You will be consuming fewer calories, which will directly impact weight loss.

2) Since you are eating WHOLE foods, you will be physically filling your stomach, reducing hunger and cravings.

3) You will be consuming less chemicals and refined ingredients such as oils with saturated fat and a host of other dangerous, carcinogenic chemicals.

4) You will start consuming WHOLE foods, which contain nutrients your body actually needs (and has been deprived of) including fiber, carbs, proteins, minerals and vitamins.

If you can do this, you will start seeing results QUICKLY and you will feel better, especially if you can couple this approach with a green smoothie each day.

You know, there are only THREE species on the planet who struggle with weight issues – one is humans, the others are cats and dogs. And what do they have in common? HUMANS!

Just as we humans make bad choices when it comes to how we eat, it's often passed onto our own pets because they depend on us for food. However, once we get a handle on this area, things can turn around rather quickly.

Every other species on the planet eats a natural diet and they THRIVE. You NEVER see an obese giraffe or a squirrel too fat to run up a tree. Animals are not just close to their ideal weight, they are PERFECTLY in shape because they eat their natural, optimal diet and, when they do, it guarantees their SURVIVAL.

PUSHING OUR LIMITS

Many believe their family genes determine whether they'll become obese, develop diabetes or even heart disease. Nothing can be further from the truth. It's like saying the next car you buy is likely to have problems because all the ones you've previously owned were trouble as well. Unless your luck with cars is just bad, the real problem is likely to be the way you've cared for or driven these vehicles than something having been destined for you.

Our genes fall into two categories, "required" and "suggested". The "required" genes we cannot control, such as our height or the color our eyes and hair. The "suggested" genes indicate we have a strong POTENTIAL for something, but we are ultimately in control of it.

For example, if your family has a history of diabetes this does not mean you are also expected to develop the disease. This indicates that, according to your genetics, if you become overweight or obese (the leading cause of diabetes) you put yourself at greater risk for becoming diabetic. Everyone has different genetic limits and our family histories remind us what they are. However, if you eat a healthy diet and maintain good health and nutritional balance, chances are you will not be susceptible to something like diabetes. This is very much like speeding in a car.

Your chances of earning a speeding ticket are directly related to not only how far you exceed the speed limit, but also how OFTEN you do so. If you speed most of the time, chances are high you'll eventually get caught. If you break the speed limit occasionally your risks are lower. However, if you NEVER speed at all, what are the chances of EVER receiving a speeding ticket?

When our genetic limits are pushed, we discover the boundaries of our health. Want to stay healthy? Don't push your own limits to find out, it's that simple.

When we live by pushing our limits, we shouldn't be surprised when history repeats itself. As a matter of fact, history is what gives us a MAJOR clue into what we SHOULD be eating.

OUR ANCESTORS ATE DIFFERENTLY THAN WE DO NOW

If you take a close look at what foods have powered our ancestors across MANY generations, you will find they also consumed large amounts of plant-based, whole foods. Specifically, I am referring to the largest civilizations on Earth who have both SURVIVED and THRIVED over long periods of time, making it possible for us to be here today.

Food	Region	Duration In Years
Barley	Middle East	11,000
Corn	North, Central, South America	7,000
Legumes (beans)	Americas, Asia, Europe	6,000
Millet	Africa	6,000
Oats	Middle East	11,000
Potatoes	South America	13,000
Rice	Asia	10,000
Wheat	Near East	10,000

Why were these plant-based foods essential to the long term survival of these many diverse civilizations? Firstly, these foods are clean, meaning they don't tend to carry viruses that are a threat to human survival such as Salmonella or E. coli. Plant-based foods are also nutritionally COMPLETE. They are packed with protein, vitamins, minerals, fiber, amino acids and carbohydrates. This is why starches such as potatoes, rice, corn and beans are commonly known as "comfort foods". They not only taste good, but are extremely SATISFYING.

Not only are plant-based foods clean, nutritious and satisfying, they also provide ENERGY. For example, the ancient Roman Gladiators consumed so much grain they have gone down in history as "the barley men". These were among the fiercest fighters on the planet and primarily fueled by plant-foods and grains. Gladiators ate this way because their survival DEPENDED on it; losing was not an option!

In modern times, look at the world's top athletes, such as Kenyans who are known to be among the healthiest, leanest, fastest endurance runners on Earth. For the past 40 years Kenyan runners have DOMINATED road running more than any other country. It's no secret that most of their nutrients come from plant-based sources and carbohydrates such as bread, boiled rice, poached potatoes, boiled porridge, cabbage, kidney beans and ugali (a corn-meal paste shaped into balls and then dipped into various foods for taste). Why do these foods work so well? Not only are these starch-based foods highly nutritious but they also provide these exceptional athletes with the sustained ENERGY needed to both COMPETE and WIN.

Aside from athletes there are CULTURES who have maintained impressive periods of health and longevity such as the Okinawans in Japan, where it is not uncommon for men to live past 100 years of age. What do they eat? Okinawans typically consume a low calorie, plant-based diet that is also low in protein and refined carbohydrates. A daily intake of 9-17 servings of vegetables, 7-13 servings of whole grains or 2-4 servings of fruit is fairly common as well. The consumption of any vegetable oils or animal-based products is fairly limited and in moderation.

Unless a plant-based food has somehow been contaminated by human beings, usually due to pesticides or improper storage, it is important to understand that fruits, vegetables and starches deliver nothing but strong, undeniable health BENEFITS. I wouldn't even know where to begin in listing ANY significant health risks from the consumption of too many plant-based, whole foods.

SECTION HIGHLIGHTS (Ch. 4)

- A food is considered "junk" when it offers little to no nutritional benefits. When we eat these foods, our body receives little nourishment – meaning we don't give ourselves much to help grow, repair or replenish blood cells or skin tissues.

- Food corporations and fast food giants have realized that by targeting our most PRIMAL taste desires they can get us to eat just about ANYTHING. Even adding items such as silly putty and wood pulp in our food by using a clever combination of the three pillars on which these companies survive – SALT, SUGAR and FAT.

- It's important to steer clear of any products containing partially hydrogenated vegetable oils, monosodium glutamate (MSG), BPA, nitrates, diacetyl, Dimethylpolysiloxane, BHT/BHA or 4-mel as they have been linked to SERIOUS, life-threatening health issues.

- Even though these chemicals are being used at levels approved "safe" by the Food & Drug Administration (FDA), these amounts have never been tested when consumed in COMBINATION and over varying lengths of time.

- A calorie is a unit of measurement. In the case of food, a calorie is a unit of ENERGY.

- One gram of carbohydrate is equal to 4 calories while one gram of fat is equal to 9 calories. We effortlessly more than DOUBLE our caloric intake when eating fattier foods.

- Foods that are high in calories but low in nutrition (vitamins, minerals, fiber, etc.) have what's known as "empty calories".

- You see, our stomachs have nutrient and stretch "sensors" which signal us once we've eaten enough food to physically fill our stomach. Once this happens we feel "full" and don't feel comfortable eating anything until our stomach empties again.

- When we eat foods that don't fill our stomach, yet supply us with high amounts of calories, we tend to overeat and, therefore, make us susceptible to weight gain.

- It's important to derive most of our calories from plant-based, whole foods which are lower in calorie, more nutrient-dense and physically fill our stomach.

- Our genes fall into two categories, "required" and "suggested". The "required" genes we cannot control, such as our height or the color our eyes and hair. The "suggested" genes indicate we have a strong POTENTIAL for something, but we are ultimately in control of it.

- The largest, most successful civilizations on Earth both survived and thrived due to the regular consumption of plant-based foods, including starches such as corn, rice, potatoes, beans and grains.

CHAPTER FIVE
Remove or Limit Dairy

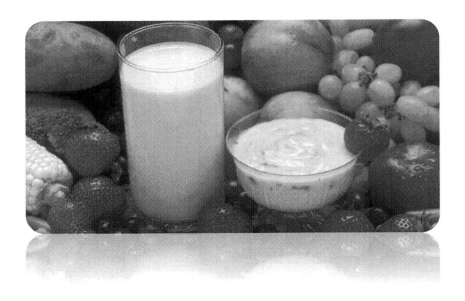

"Did you know humans are the only species on the planet who drink the milk of another species? We are also the ONLY species who continue drinking milk after our infancy."

DAIRY PRODUCTS INCLUDE

Milk, eggs, cheese, butter, yogurt, cottage cheese, kefir, ice cream, milkshakes, sour cream and more.

At the beginning of this book I claimed we are all being POISONED. However, it's not just our food that contains toxins, but our MIND as well. We are being poisoned with bad INFORMATION that, in turn, leads us to make poor health decisions. Imagine being advised by someone you trusted to use diesel instead of gasoline as fuel in your car... and you believe them! What kind of damage would that do to your engine?

The dairy industry actually has people believing that a product such as cow's milk is one of the best ways "to ensure your diet is nutritious and balanced". They also claim we need milk for calcium to build stronger bones. Have you ever stopped to think where the calcium in milk actually comes from? Calcium is a MINERAL and originates from the SOIL. Cows get it from the plants they eat. If cows get their calcium from plants, why do we need to get our calcium filtered through the udder of a cow? Simple, we don't. Plus, the high acidity of dairy causes our bones to release sulfur in order to neutralize the acid, weakening them in the process and increasing our risk of osteoporosis.

As a matter of fact, believing we need cow's milk for ANY reason is completely misleading. *Did you know humans are the ONLY species on the planet who drink the milk of another species? We are also the ONLY species who continue drinking milk after our infancy.* How could we have possibly gotten this so wrong? Again, we have a multi-million dollar dairy industry that needs to sell PRODUCT and therefore convince you it's something you absolutely need. It's just "Business 101".

When you further understand the role of mother's milk for any mammal species, this becomes even clearer. For example, human breast milk is ESSENTIAL for human babies during the most crucial time of their lives, when nervous, respiratory and immune systems are being strengthened. Human breast milk contains just the right amount of protein and other nutrients to ensure infants are properly nourished and grown to a particular size during this very important time.

Similarly, cow's milk contains just the right nutrient density and growth hormones to grow a baby calf from 60 lbs. to 600 lbs. in six months; in other words, LARGE growth over a SHORT period of time. This applies to ALL mammals on the planet – the breast milk produced for their babies is *tailored to their species* for its own growth requirements and they NEVER drink it again for the rest of their lives.

What has been the cost to human health by over consumption of cow's milk and its derived products, namely cheese, butter and other dairy?

OBESITY

There are a couple of key reasons why people are now more overweight than ever. One of them is due to the regular consumption of fat and growth hormones (animal proteins) naturally occurring in dairy products. For example, cheese is about 70% fat by nature and found in many of the foods we eat regularly. According to the USDA, in 1909 the average person consumed less than 4lbs of cheese per year. Today, each American consumes around 33lbs per year! So what has caused this dramatic change in our eating habits?

In the 1950s we witnessed the rise of fast food chains and TV dinners and shortly afterwards, junk foods such as flavored snack chips. Eventually, people could pick up a phone and have these foods delivered right to their door! At first we treated these convenient food options more as delicacies, only indulging as time or money allowed. Today, however, our lives are seemingly CENTERED on where to go eat and finding quick foods at the grocery store that are cheap and easy to make. In the process *we have sacrificed quality for convenience.* We gradually began DISCONNECTING from our mostly plant-based eating habits that once made us strong and more towards poor decisions that have weakened us and wreaked havoc on our health.

What happens when we are overweight or obese? As I mentioned earlier, an environment is created inside our body that promotes disease. One of the biggest diseases related to obesity is Type-2 diabetes. Many will tell you this disease is caused by eating too much sugar, which is not true. As I mentioned earlier, sugar (or glucose) is VITAL to every single cell in our body, which use it as the primary source of FUEL.

The way sugar enters our cells is by insulin, which is secreted by the pancreas. However, when our cells get too fatty the insulin becomes ineffective at allowing the sugar inside, known as "insulin resistance". Once this happens the excess sugar remains in our blood supply, causing blood sugar levels to dramatically rise. A doctor will give us medication to reduce our blood sugar levels; however, this does not solve the problem, it only helps us live WITH it. In most cases, this disease can be REVERSED by simply losing weight. As we learned earlier, this is done by consuming less fat calories, specifically, staying away from foods with saturated fat which caused our cells to become fatty in the first place.

When we have an environment inside our body that PROMOTES disease it is like losing that bodyguard I talked about earlier. Once this happens, we're vulnerable to not only heart disease and diabetes but a host of MANY other health problems.

COMMON ILLNESS

When we consume a food considered FOREIGN to our body there is a natural reaction against it. Perhaps you've heard of "lactose intolerance". This is a condition directly related to the consumption of dairy products causing bloating, cramps, diarrhea, flatulence, nausea, rumbling stomach and vomiting. You see, humans naturally lose the enzyme responsible for properly digesting the lactose in milk after infancy. This causes "lactose intolerance" for many who continue drinking milk after nature's plan is complete.

Most people are affected and don't even realize it, *especially Asian and African Americans, who are estimated to be 70-90% affected by this disorder.* The way to improve lactose intolerance is to simply remove dairy from ones diet, or in other words, *stop eating the foods we shouldn't be eating in the first place.*

When we center our everyday meals on these rich, allergenic foods is it any wonder Americans are struggling with so many health issues? When we consume foods that work AGAINST us, it leads to a host of common illnesses that have us frequently running to the doctor including stomach cramps, diarrhea, sinus infections, asthma, arthritis, lupus, acne, hyperactivity, fatigue, depression, anemia, to name just a few.

The chart below confirms various characteristics of dairy products (milk, cheese, butter, eggs) and the health risks they pose to humans due to regular consumption:

Associated with Dairy	Increased Risks Include...
Highly Allergenic	Autoimmune allergies (arthritis, lupus, type-1 diabetes), lactose intolerance
Microbes, organisms	Infectious disease
Environmental contaminants (DDT, PCB)	Cancer, Parkinson's Disease, hormone imbalance
High calorie High saturated fat	Obesity, type-2 diabetes, heart disease, cancer
High Protein	Kidney damage, kidney stones, osteoporosis
Highly Acidic	Osteoporosis, kidney stones
High Cholesterol	Heart disease, strokes, heart attacks
Low Iron	Anemia, iron deficiency
No dietary fiber	Constipation

The bacterium, microbes and growth hormones inherently found in dairy products is just scratching the surface. Here are some other startling findings I uncovered while researching dairy:

- The USDA does not allow ANY company or advertisement to claim eggs are "nutritious", "healthy" or even "safe". This is because a single egg is 67% FAT and has over 212mg of cholesterol, not to mention, over 100,000 Americans die each year from salmonella poisoning. Now, you will hear MANY experts and health gurus emphatically claim, "Eggs are good for you!" However, if the USDA can't even stake that claim, how can THEY?

- A SINGLE egg contains more cholesterol than a Hardee's Thickburger. Excessive amounts of dietary cholesterol is the main reason why people are diagnosed with "high cholesterol" and, therefore, at a higher risk of heart disease.

- According to a 2003 report, 40% of all beef herds and 64% of dairy herds in the USA are infected with the Bovine Aids Virus (BIV) and 89% of dairy herds are infected with the Bovine Leukemia Virus (BLV). This means you can pretty much count on viruses, even in small amounts, present in most milk and dairy products. How do these animals get infected? Many are sharing the same syringe for medications, tattooing or dehorning instruments and, in many cases, it's simply passed from mother to calf. This is nothing new, however. It's been well established that our meat and dairy herds have been infected with viruses since as early as 1969. Do you think there is any correlation between the consumption of foods containing leukemia antibodies and the 150,000+ who will be diagnosed with leukemia this year? How about the fact that every three minutes in the USA someone is diagnosed with having blood cancer?

- The growth hormones naturally occurring in dairy products can lead to the early onset of puberty in girls as well as large breasts at a very early age.

- Since dairy cows virtually become "milking machines" they are given added growth hormones to increase milk production. This often makes them become seriously ill with various diseases, including mastitis, an infection of the udder that ultimately contaminates milk with PUS. But don't worry; the FDA has set a "safe level" of pus per glass! In more technical terms, one CC (cubic centimeter) of cow's milk is allowed to have 750,000 somatic cells (white blood cells, or "pus").

- It's not just our food that contains toxins, but our MIND as well. We are being poisoned with bad INFORMATION that, in turn, leads us to make poor health decisions.

- Humans are the ONLY species on the planet who drink the milk of another species. We are also the ONLY species who continue drinking milk after our infancy.

- Mother's milk is tailored to each species to ensure proper nutrition so as to grown a baby to a certain size over a particular period of time.

- The dairy industry needs to sell a PRODUCT and have people believing they need cow's milk for calcium to build stronger bones.

- Calcium is a MINERAL and comes from the PLANTS which cows eat.

- Dairy products such as milk, cheese and butter are "rich" foods and contain large amounts of saturated fat, cholesterol and animal proteins, which fuel growth (obesity or puberty in young girls) and can lead to common health conditions and diseases.

- Obesity is the main cause of Type-2 Diabetes. This occurs when insulin loses its ability to allow sugar into our blood cells because they have become too "fatty".

- When we consume a food considered FOREIGN to our body there is a natural reaction against it. Lactose intolerance is a health disorder that affects most people and they don't realize it.

- Most dairy in the USA is infected with varying amounts of either BIV (Bovine Aids Virus) or BLV (Bovine Leukemia Virus) and has been since at least the late 60's.

- The USDA does not allow ANY company to claim eggs are "nutritious", "healthy" or even "safe" for human consumption.

CHAPTER SIX
Remove or Limit Meat Consumption

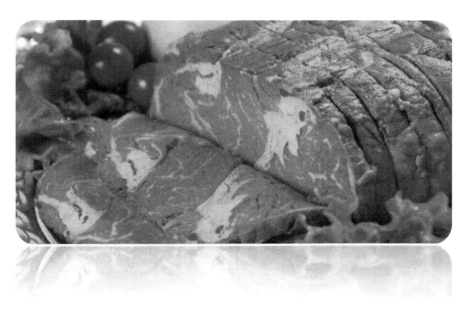

"No civilization on the planet has EVER consumed animal foods in the amounts that we do today. As expected, the results are a society with never before seen epidemic health problems."

Let's ask ourselves an honest question…

If we couldn't walk into a grocery store or restaurant to either buy or order beef, chicken, pork or fish, how much would that change our consumption of those foods?

Even if you possessed hunting skills you would likely eat a MODERATE amount considering how much time and effort it takes to produce even a single meal. Of course, if you had no hunting skills at all, you are not likely to consume any meat whatsoever.

This is because, left to our own devices, humans are instinctively not designed to detect, chase, kill or even digest animal flesh very efficiently. We don't have heightened senses of hearing, sight or smell to find prey very easily. We're not very fast runners compared to wild animals and don't possess razor sharp claws or teeth to tear into and chew through raw flesh. Naysayers often claim to have "canine teeth". I say to them, open your cat or dog's mouth and look inside. Now, compare it to what's in your mouth – not even close.

When it comes to digestion, we have very lengthy intestines where meat not only takes long to pass through but often never makes it out and winds up rotting in our digestive tract.

When you think about it, if humans were INSTINCTIVELY designed to eat meat we are at a SEVERE disadvantage from every other species on this planet that ARE designed to eat meat, known as carnivores. Not surprisingly we have MUCH more in common with the species that instinctively eat plant-based foods, known as herbivores.

Carnivores	Herbivores	Humans
Has claws	No claws	No claws
No pores, perspires through tongue, "panting"	Perspires through pores on skin, sweating	Perspires through pores on skin, sweating
Sharp, pointed front teeth	No sharp, pointed front teeth	No sharp, pointed front teeth, flattened.
Acidic saliva, no enzyme to pre-digest carbohydrates	Alkaline saliva, enzymes to pre-digest carbohydrates	Alkaline saliva, enzymes to pre-digest carbohydrates
Strong hydrochloric stomach acid to digest meat, bone, etc.	Stomach acid 20 times weaker than carnivores.	Stomach acid 20 times weaker than carnivores.
Intestinal tract is 3 times body length for rapid release of food.	Intestinal tract is 10-12 (or more) times body length for much longer release of food.	Intestinal tract is 10-12 (or more) times body length for much longer release of food.
Mouth opening vs head size is large.	Mouth opening vs head size is small.	Mouth opening vs head size is small.
Jaws have no side-to side motion, "shearing" action.	Jaws have good side-to side motion, no "shearing" action.	Jaws have good side-to side motion, no "shearing" action.

When we take a closer look at how we instinctively react to certain foods, it clearly defines the way we're meant to eat. For example, when we see a dead animal by the side of road, or ANYWHERE for that matter, do we automatically get hungry or begin eating the flesh right off the bone? Of course not, to us that is disgusting. However a dog, cat, bear, fox or raccoon would gladly dig right in because, instinctively, that is THEIR food.

What happens when we see an apple, a salad or bowl of mashed potatoes? We feel a primal connection with those foods and would not hesitate to eat them as is. Why? This is because fruits, vegetables and carbohydrates are OUR food.

Does this mean we can NEVER eat meat? No, of course not. Humans have eaten meat through much of our history. For some it was a means of survival, for others a mere delicacy. However, no civilization on the planet has EVER consumed animal foods in the amounts that we do today.

After all the research I've done and realizing the health risks closely associated with meat, dairy and highly processed foods, I believe animal foods should be treated as DELICACIES at best due to their RICH nature. These foods contain high concentrations of saturated fat, cholesterol, growth hormones, microbes, bacteria, chemicals and potential viruses. Eating too much of these foods has proven DEVASTATING on human health. If only we learned to either greatly reduce or remove these foods from our diet entirely, we would see much improvement to both our short term and long term health.

When it comes to our own health, the more we deprive our body of what it ACTUALLY needs to run optimally, the greater our risk of introducing trouble. As we've seen, trouble can come in many ways, including clogging our arteries.

HEART DISEASE

Certain foods cause irritation, inflammation, leave behind residues and promote the growth of plaque inside our arteries. Over time, a buildup of too much plaque leads to those arteries getting clogged up. Every time we consume foods rich in cholesterol and saturated fat, we are increasing the risk of clogging the arteries inside our body. If the artery leads to our heart, it's known as a heart attack; if the artery leads to our brain, it's a stroke; if you're a man and the artery goes "downstairs", it's called "erectile dysfunction" (or E.D). As a matter of fact, E.D. is the "canary in the coalmine", meaning if that artery is having issues, chances are good the same is happening elsewhere.

Another early indicator of heart disease is a condition known as "high blood pressure". This happens when our heart has to exert more pressure to get the blood moving through our arteries due to an obstruction. Have you ever seen a gutter blocked by so many leaves that it overflows with rainwater? Obviously the best way to prevent this is to keep the gutter free from any leaves in the first place. The arteries within our body act much the same way. The more our arteries are kept clean and clear, the easier our blood can flow and therefore guarantee a heart attack or stroke is not likely to happen.

So where do we find cholesterol and saturated fats? Look no further than ALL animal and dairy related products, including vegetable oils such as beef, chicken, pork, fish, eggs, milk, cheese, butter or olive oil. Does this mean if we eat a few eggs or hamburgers we will get a heart attack? Of course not, but that is the problem.

The buildup of plaque in one's arteries takes time just as the drain in your bathtub doesn't clog overnight. It is a slow, gradual buildup of hair and other things that eventually prevents the water in your tub from draining out. When your tub clogs, you add a chemical to fix the problem. When it's your heart that's clogged, you go under a knife and then directed to take medications for the rest of your life. This is why heart disease, stroke and high blood pressure are known as "silent killers" because they often take YEARS before you get the first symptoms, or worse, an "attack".

Now, some will argue that humans have been consuming meat and dairy for many thousands of years and that if it was so damaging to our health, we wouldn't have survived as a species. However, our ancestors did not consume these foods anywhere CLOSE to the amounts we do in modern times.

Our ancestors did not have grocery stores or fast food drive-thrus on most street corners or a meat and dairy industry RELENTLESSLY promoting their products as "essential" to our health. You see even though tobacco smoking, as we know it today, has been around since the 1700's, it wasn't until the 1970's that scientific evidence proved convincingly that smoking was bad for our health and promoted lung cancer. Even though the tobacco industry still does well, they suffered a MAJOR financial setback due to the stigma associated with their unhealthy product.

The meat and dairy industry took notice and vowed this would NOT happen to them, even in light of strong evidence their products contain ingredients that promote heart disease, diabetes and most all of our killer diseases. These industries have a CONSIDERABLE amount of money, power and influence at play inside our government and work tirelessly to not only suppress hard evidence revealing their products in a negative light but also to promote them as essential to our health and well-being.

True, our ancestors ate animal products from time to time, especially in extreme situations, but nothing that compares with today's consumption levels. As a matter of fact, the only real example of a predominantly meat eating culture were the Inuit Eskimos. They lived on the extremes, in a very cold climate where the cultivation of plant foods for any length of time was not feasible. What was the result? The Inuit survived almost exclusively on meat, lived an average of 27 years and were found to have had massive heart disease.

Today, we live in a culture where it's common to have bacon and eggs for breakfast, ham and cheese with milk for lunch, maybe a yogurt in the afternoon, a steak or hamburger for dinner and then perhaps a snack afterwards with even more milk and dairy. Never in human history have large civilizations EVER eaten like this! Today, it's common to CENTER all our meals on meat and dairy products and, as expected, the results are a society with never before seen epidemic health problems. Heart disease is the #1 killer among Americans and has held that distinction for DECADES.

CANCER

Every single one of us has cells in our bodies capable of becoming cancerous. How well these good cells are able to mutate, develop their own blood vessels, multiply and become a threat to our health depends on how well we are taking care of the INSIDE of our body. One of the biggest problems with consuming animal products are they introduce all sorts of microbes and bacteria into our tissues and blood supply. And why should that be surprising? Let's be honest, we ARE talking about the consumption of rotting flesh, regardless of the source.

According to the February 2014 issue of Consumer Reports, 97% of the chicken they randomly tested from grocery stores in the United States was CONTAMINATED with salmonella. *Even though salmonella bacteria are mostly killed off during the cooking process, they still contaminate kitchen counters and utensils used in food preparation* and remain a serious health threat after the meal has ended. How many times have you ever heard of major beef recalls due to E. coli contamination? Just do a Google search on "beef recalls" and you will easily see how meat is recalled on a monthly basis across the country mainly due to contamination from bacteria. Quite simply, *most meat of ANY kind is full of bacteria, microbes and potential viruses, which is EXACTLY what triggers normal cells to become malignant, or cancerous.*

Remember earlier how I mentioned cow's milk is designed to grow a baby calf at a fast rate over a short period of time? *This is because dairy naturally contains growth factors that FUEL the rapid growth of ALL cells – both healthy and cancerous.*

Just as there is a "symphony" of foods and ingredients that work WITH our body in promoting good health, there is another "symphony" that does the opposite. The chart below confirms various characteristics of meat (beef, chicken, pork & fish) and the health risks they pose to humans due to regular consumption:

Associated with Meat	Increased Risks Include...
Low Iron	Infectious disease, cancer
Naturally occurring microbes, organisms, bacteria, salmonella, e. coli	Cancer, Parkinson's Disease, hormone imbalance
Environmental contaminants (DDT, PCB), Bio-magnification, mercury (fish)	Cancer
Carcinogens from cooking	Constipation
High calorie, High saturated fat	Obesity, type-2 diabetes, heart disease
High Protein	Kidney damage, kidney stones, osteoporosis
Highly Acid	Osteoporosis, kidney stones
High Cholesterol, Saturated Fat	Heart disease, strokes, heart attacks
Associated with Meat	Increased Risks Include...
No Carbohydrate	Fatigue
No Calcium/Vitamin C	Poor Tissues
No dietary fiber	Constipation

Earlier I talked about testing our hereditary limits. Below are the Top 15 killers in America for 2014, a result of pushing our own genetic limits:

1. Heart Disease
2. Alzheimer's
3. Suicide
4. Cancer
5. Diabetes
6. Liver Disease
7. Stroke
8. Influenza and Pneumonia
9. Hypertension
10. Lung Disease
11. Kidney Disease
12. Parkinson's
13. Accidents
14. Blood Poisoning
15. Homicide

All of the diseases shown above are linked to poor dietary choices. These are exactly the types of diseases that are encouraged to develop when our internal environment is not geared for good health and we push our hereditary limits.

Simply put, when we center our diets on plant-based, whole foods we greatly REDUCE our risk of ever having these sorts of problems. *When it comes to heart disease, our #1 killer, you can literally become heart attack proof simply by changing how you eat. It IS that simple.* If you already have some of these problems, chances are it's not too late to begin reversing them TODAY by eating a diet that PROTECTS and FIGHTS against disease instead of one that INVITES it.

Now, you could go the route most people take in treating these types of diseases with prescribed medications. You'll find one pill to lower your cholesterol, another to reduce blood sugar or yet another for blood pressure. However, simply centering your meals on more natural, plant-based foods will take care of it all without drugs.

While Americans comprise of only 5% of the world's population, we consume 50% of ALL pharmaceutical drugs. Prescription drugs kill more than 100,000 Americans each year. These deaths are not from misuse, abuse or overdoses; just from side effects alone. If we factored this into the chart above, "death by medication" would come in at #6. Even if someone doesn't die from prescription pills, the toxic load of these medications on our body is devastating over time and often leads to decreased quality of life. *Simply put, medications will rarely if ever cure you of anything and merely prolong what you already have. Eating plant-based, whole foods trump medicine EVERY time when fighting disease.*

Sadly, medicine and sickness is a BUSINESS that is more interested in your money than your health. If pills worked, America would be leading the world in reversed diseases. Have you ever seen a television advertisement for prescription medications?

They spend the first few seconds telling you just how GREAT their product is! You see images of happy people smiling warmly at the camera, going about their day. Then, while that's happening, the second half of the ad warns how this wonderful pill can cause dizziness, trouble breathing, ulcers, liver failure, hemorrhages, an increased risk of stroke, even thoughts of suicide! If this doesn't spell it all out for you, perhaps we need to look a little closer to home.

OUR KIDS TELL THE STORY

If you really need MORE evidence as to what is compromising our health, look no further than our children. One of the most alarming health epidemics in America is the increasingly poor health of our youth.

Nearly ALL children have begun developing fatty streaks in their arteries by the age of 10, otherwise known as the beginning stages of heart disease. More than 1/3 of all children are obese. Type-2 diabetes, a disease previously found only in adults over 40, is becoming more common among children. One in three children in America has high cholesterol. Why is this happening?

Quite simply, *children are adopting the same poor eating habits that are getting their parents in the SAME trouble; only kids are getting a much EARLIER start.* If that's not enough, every time they turn on a television they're constantly bombarded with billions of advertising dollars promoting fast food, junk food and all sorts of cholesterol and saturated fatty products as "all natural" and "healthy".

An alarming 84% of American parents admit to feeding their children fast food at least once a week. For anyone who STILL does not believe that meat, dairy and other highly concentrated, "rich" products such as fried foods and sodas are not to blame, they really need to ask themselves this question – WHAT IS?

When you watch the footage of an open heart surgery you can see the surgeon pulling out plaque from an artery. That is not a Brussels sprout or green bean – it is FAT. And *just as there is a symphony of healthy foods that nourish our bodies, there is another symphony of foods that triggers disease.*

If we want to protect ourselves, our family and loved ones from becoming an alarming statistic, it is time to look closely at how we eat and decide how we can begin making changes TODAY.

SECTION HIGHLIGHTS (Ch. 6)

- The meat and dairy industry have products to sell and mislead you with false health benefit claims.

- We do not need to consume cow's milk for calcium.

- We can get our calcium from the same place cows get theirs, from plants.

- Dairy products are "rich" foods, containing high amounts of saturated fat and cholesterol.
- Obesity is the main cause of Type-2 Diabetes.

- When we consume products our body considers "foreign" we have natural reactions.

- Lactose intolerance is a health disorder that affects most people and they don't realize it.

- The USDA will not allow any company to claim eggs are "nutritious", "healthy" or even "safe".

- Meat of any kind contains cholesterol and saturated fat which are the main triggers of heart disease.

- Meat contains bacteria, microbes and often viruses that trigger cancer.

- When cooked, meat contains carcinogens that can trigger cancer growth as well as other health issues.

- The common solution for treating illness is prescription drugs, which not only kill over 100,000 people per year but rarely address the root cause of any health issue.

- Children in America are becoming unhealthier with over 1/3 considered obese, most developing fatty streaks in their arteries by age 10 and type-2 diabetes reaching epidemic levels.

CHAPTER SEVEN
How to Shop Healthy

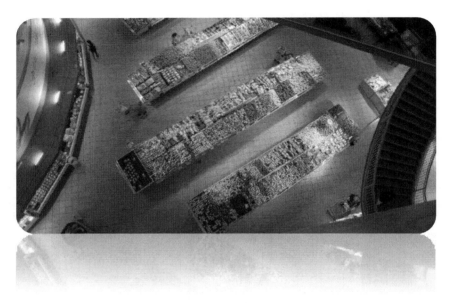

"Ever seen the words "all-natural", "fat-free", "made with real fruit", "sugar free" or even "organic" used to promote a product? These are all TRICKS to make you think the product is a healthier choice than it actually is."

Some say healthy eating begins with what we put in our mouth. I say it starts with what we put in our shopping cart because, ultimately, that's what we wind up bringing home and eating. It's what we decide to eat for breakfast, lunch, midday snack, dinner or what we reach for late at night after getting "the munchies". Too often if we've made poor choices at the grocery store, we continue them in the heat of a hungry moment. This is why it's important to make wise, healthy decisions at the store so that we can do the same at home.

Let's recap the low-risk, healthy, plant-based foods which we should be centering our meals around:

Fruits	Berries, apples, oranges, pears, melons, grapes, bananas, figs, mangoes, peaches, pineapples, dates, cherries.
Vegetables	Spinach, kale, celery, carrots, broccoli, artichokes, peppers, squash, lettuce, Brussels sprouts, cabbage, onions, cauliflower.
Starches	Potatoes, sweet potatoes.
Grains	Oats, barley, wheat, buckwheat, millet, rice, corn, whole grain pasta, quinoa (a seed).
Legumes	Beans, peas, lentils.

Now that you've learned more about which foods are high and low risk, your trips to the grocery store can be faster, more efficient and less-expensive than ever before. *Just remember that most of the products in any given grocery store are useless to a healthy diet.* Knowing this will cut down your browse time and grocery bill considerably.

Some may suggest shopping the perimeter of the grocery store. However, I believe those areas contain some of the most unhealthiest foods, rich in cholesterol and saturated fat, such as milk, eggs, cheese and meats. While you'll find fruits, vegetables and potatoes along the perimeter of most any store, starches such as rice, beans and grains are likely to be found in the middle aisles.

Also, it would be a good idea to become acquainted with how your grocery store handles certified organic products. Do they have a dedicated area for organic foods or are they mixed in with conventional products? Many stores do a combination of both.

BEFORE MAKING RADICAL CHANGES

After reading this book you may feel like you have to start making MAJOR changes to how you're shopping and eating and begin buying foods you aren't familiar with. Before we go any further, please understand this is NOT the best way to proceed.

If you only change ONE thing about the way you're currently eating, you are on the right path. For example, if you only add one green smoothie to your day, you will be better off than before. If you stop consuming soda and begin drinking spring water, that is another little victory. Instead of ordering from a drive-thru three times a week, cut it back to once a week – this is all PROGRESS.

The more you begin introducing healthy, plant-based, whole foods into your diet and can remove something of risk, the more nutritionally balanced you will become. Once you begin noticing how much better you both look and feel, the more you will want to further tweak the way you eat.

Whether your goal is to lose weight or simply be healthier, it all starts at the grocery store. Below I will share some tips on how to simply look at a product and determine how healthy a choice it actually is.

USDA ORGANIC vs. CONVENTIONAL PRODUCTS

Are organic foods really that much better than conventional ones? It depends on what you're buying. Often people equate the USDA Organic seal with "healthy", no matter what it's found on. You can buy a bag of organic potato chips, cookies or even breakfast cereal, but that doesn't necessarily save you from consuming empty calories or high amounts of saturated fat. And certainly when it comes to meat or dairy products, organic doesn't remove the cholesterol, saturated fat or inherent growth hormones, which are major contributors to heart disease, obesity, cancer and many other health issues.

The major thing to understand about the USDA Organic certification is that an additional set of standards are in place which go above and beyond those in conventional products. For example, instead of using chemical fertilizers or synthetic pesticides, certified organic farmers must use only natural fertilizers such as manure or compost. On animal farms, the use of antibiotics or added growth hormones are prohibited and animals must be raised on organic feed and have access to the outdoors.

When you buy certified organic, you're simply REDUCING health risks by consuming foods free of both artificial pesticides and ingredients more than anything else. Organic doesn't always guarantee healthier, even if it's a fruit or vegetable. The differences between organic and conventional produce, in terms of nutrients, is insignificant, at best. However, anytime you can buy food that has fewer added chemicals or contaminants, such as pesticides, and held to a higher production standard, the better.

The Vital Blend's Organic vs. Conventional		
(based on USDA Standards)	ORGANIC	CONVENTIONAL
Toxic Persistent Pesticides	Not Allowed	Allowed
GMOs	Not Allowed	Allowed
Antibiotics	Not Allowed	Allowed
Growth Hormones	Not Allowed	Allowed
Sludge and Irradiation	Not Allowed	Allowed
Animal Welfare Requirements	Yes	No
Cows Required To Be On Pasture For Pasture Season	Yes	No
Lower Levels Of Environmental Pollution	Yes	Not Necessary
Audit Trail From Farm To Table	Yes	No
Certifications Required, Including Inspections	Yes	No
Legal Restrictions On Allowable Materials	Yes	No

WHAT ABOUT GLUTEN FREE?

When it comes to gluten free ANYTHING just remember that, for the most part, this is another type of food label that people often associate with "healthy". The only ones who really need to be concerned with gluten free foods are those suffering from a condition known as "celiac disease". Those struggling with this disease experience adverse reactions including skin rashes, muscular problems or digestive issues. There is no mistaking someone who is allergic to gluten; however, this condition only affects about 1 in 100 people. Unfortunately, it's become more of a "fad" and now many believe it's something they also need to be concerned with.

If you have celiac disease, or perhaps chronic diarrhea (or irritable bowel syndrome), stay with "gluten free" products. Otherwise, don't be overly concerned about foods carrying this label. As a matter of fact, gluten is often beneficial as it helps grow the good bacteria in our gut. As with ANY food, if you eat something and feel bad as a result, stop eating it.

WHAT ABOUT GMO's?

So, what are GMOs? It stands for "genetically modified organisms". Remember in the first chapter when I spoke about our human DNA? Well, plants have DNA too. Back in the 1990's scientists found a way to alter a plant's DNA so it could do things normal plants couldn't.

For example, if a crop of corn was becoming decimated by insects, scientists would "splice in" DNA from bacteria or viruses so when a bug ate it, their stomach would explode. This genetic modification would also allow farmers to spray more pesticides without harming the crop. What effect does this have on humans? Quite simply, we don't know for sure and that is the problem.

When it comes to labeling such foods know that, currently, there is no legal requirement for a GMO product or ingredient to be labeled in the USA. Any "Non-GMO" labels you see on products are completely voluntary. As a matter of fact, the companies who produce GMO products, such as Monsanto, have loads of money, power and influence within our government to see things remain this way. Why? What do they have to hide? What do they stand to lose by placing an honest label on their products?

Because this area is so shady and unclear, it's a good idea to stay away from GMOs period. While GMOs have been in our food supply since the late 1990s, there has yet to be a reputable scientific study showing CONCLUSIVELY that GMOs are harmful to humans. However, the companies responsible for these products do not have our best health interests in mind, only their own profits.

The chart below is a list of the most commonly genetically modified foods in the USA. To avoid GMOs in these products, buy "USDA Certified Organic" as regulations prohibit their use:

Corn *	Soy *	Yellow Crookneck Squash and Zucchini	Alfalfa
Canola *	Sugar Beets *	Cotton *	Papaya
(*) also found in soybean oil, cottonseed oil, canola oil, citric acids and corn syrups.			

PACKAGED FOODS

Packaged foods are simply those already packed in a container, typically made of cardboard or plastic and contain an ingredient list, along with nutritional information. These are also known as "convenience foods" since, in some cases all they require is you open, heat and serve. *While not all packaged foods in America are unhealthy, around 80% of them contain ingredients that have been BANNED in other countries.* For example, some of our popular breakfast cereals include such chemicals as butylated hydroxyanisole (BHA) and butylated hydroxytoluene (BHT) which are made from petroleum, a known cancer-causing agent. These chemicals have been BANNED for use in foods over in England and Japan but are FDA approved in the USA.

This shouldn't be totally surprising when you remember that food companies will add just about ANYTHING into their food these days to cut costs while continuing to claim "all-natural" on the front of the packaging. Of course the best way to KNOW if something is "all-natural" is to simply ask yourself, "did this product come from the ground"? You can safely answer "no" to most anything found in a bag, container, or box.

Remember that when you are eating anything less than a WHOLE, natural food, the missing ingredients have been replaced with SOMETHING. These replacement ingredients (often chemicals) are added to maintain color, flavor or even texture.

When you're in a grocery store and staring at a boxed food, here are some quick guidelines to make your decisions faster and healthier:

Don't Believe Any Claims Made on the Front of the Packaging

The front of any packaged food is much like a billboard or advertisement in a magazine. This space is the "canvas" where advertisers try hooking you on their products, often by using clever, misleading phrases and claims. Ever seen the words "all-natural", "fat free", "made with real fruit", "sugar free" or even "organic" used to promote a product? These are all TRICKS to make you think the product is a healthier choice than it actually is.

For example, a product like milk could say "2% fat" on the carton but that doesn't mean it only contains 2% fat. What they are not telling you is, by WEIGHT, the entire carton contains 2% fat. But who drinks milk by total weight? While an entire carton of milk may contain 2% fat, 35% of its CALORIES are from FAT. To put perspective on this, an 8oz. glass of whole milk has as much saturated fat as four strips of bacon. As for claims such as "all-natural", there is NO legal standard for the term "natural" according to the FDA, so it can be used however a company sees fit. A product can even claim to be "organic" but unless it shows the USDA Organic Logo, it's as organic as Cap'n Crunch.

READING PRODUCT LABELS

The most important parts of ANY packaged food are the *Ingredients List* and *Nutrition Facts*; all other claims, you can pretty much ignore:

Ingredients List

Before examining the nutritional information, check to see what is actually exactly IN the product. Often, just by scanning the ingredients you can tell if something is healthy or not. First, notice how LONG the ingredients list is. If it looks like a paragraph out of a novel, be wary. The longer the list, the more PROCESSING went into making the product. More processing usually means LESS natural ingredients and MORE chemicals or food substitutes were used to create the product.

Ideally, an ingredient list should only have a handful of things, at most. For example, if you're buying maple syrup, the ingredients should say "maple syrup"; Oatmeal should say "rolled oats". If you were to pick up a package of flavored, instant oats, you're likely to see a much longer ingredient list with "caramel coloring", not so "natural" flavorings as well as added sugar and salt. Some items, such as spaghetti sauce, will require more than a single ingredient but the main things to watch out for are words such as "high fructose corn syrup" (or any "corn syrups"), "hydrogenated oil", "monosodium glutamate (MSG)", "Yellow #", "Blue #", "natural flavors", "caramel color", "enriched" or "bleached".

Below are examples of good and bad ingredient labels. The worst offenders are noted in **bold italic** below:

Food	Poor Ingredient List	Preferred Ingredient List
Packaged Pasta	Semolina (Wheat), Durum Flour (Wheat), **Modified Wheat Starch**, Wheat Gluten, Niacin, Ferrous Sulfate (Iron), Thiamin Mononitrate, Riboflavin, Folic Acid.	Organic Durum Wheat Semolina (or best if the word "whole" appears *first* in the list)
Ketchup	Tomato Concentrate from Red Ripe Tomatoes, Distilled Vinegar, **High Fructose Corn Syrup, Corn Syrup**, Salt, Spice, Onion Powder, **Natural Flavoring**.	Organic tomato concentrate (water, organic tomato paste), organic sugar, organic vinegar, salt, organic onion powder, organic spices
Oatmeal	Whole Grain Rolled Oats, Calcium Carbonate, Salt, Guar Gum, **Carmel Color**, Reduced Iron, Vitamin A Palmitate.	Rolled Oats.
Peanut Butter	Roasted Peanuts, Sugar, **Hydrogenated Vegetable oils (cottonseed, soybean and rapeseed)** to prevent separation, salt.	Organic roasted peanuts, contains 1% or less of salt.

Nutrition Facts

When it comes to the Nutrition Facts label there are only FOUR key areas you really need to pay close attention to: *Serving Size, Calories from Fat, Fiber* and *Cholesterol*. Other areas will contain information that's nice to know and useful as a guide and some information is just plain useless.

MOST IMPORTANT

Serving Size – Take note of the recommended serving size. This is what ALL the numbers below are based on. You need to see if this is a realistic serving size for YOU. If not, determine what is and then multiply the numbers accordingly. For example, if one serving of rolled oats is a ½ cup, does that sound like the amount you would eat? If one cup is more like it, you will need to double all the numbers you see below. If one serving is 4g of fat and you double the serving size, you're really consuming 8g. The serving size gets trickier as you purchase more heavily processed foods. For example, if you buy a frozen pizza one serving is likely to be 1/3 of the entire pie. If you will be eating the WHOLE pie yourself, multiple all the numbers related to fat, calories, etc. by three and take note.

Calories from Fat - Earlier I discussed how calories from fat are more than DOUBLE than those from carbohydrates. For this reason, it's important to know how many of the calories you're consuming are derived from fat. *A good rule of thumb is to make sure no more than 20% of the calories you're eating per serving come from fat.* For example, if a product has 310 calories per serving and 90 of those calories come from fat, it means 30% of the calories from each serving are fat.

Below is an example of two types of Macaroni and Cheese:

Brand	Cal.	Calories From Fat	% of calories from fat	Better Option
Rob's Mac N' Cheese	310	93	30%	No
Chloe's Macaroni and Cheese	270	40	15%	Yes

In the example above, *Chloe's Macaroni and Cheese* is the better option because it contains half as much fat per serving than *Rob's Mac N' Cheese*.

While current nutrition labels in the United States clearly identify "Calories from Fat", the newly proposed label, unfortunately, does NOT. To get around this, simply multiply the grams of fat shown by 9 (or 10 if that's easier) and you will have the estimated calories from fat. For example, if a product has 4 grams of fat, multiply it by 9 and you'll know 36 of its calories are from fat. To then determine the percentage of calories from fat, take the total number of calories and multiply by .2 (or 20%). Is the result equal to or less than the total number of calories from fat? If so, you have determined this food is actually LOW in fat.

For example, if a product has 190 calories and 36 are from fat, multiply 190 by .2 and you get 38. With the product having 36 calories from fat, this means it is just under 20% fat. If your result was 40 or a little higher it doesn't mean you can't eat it, just be AWARE that you're eating something that contains more than 20% fat per serving. Consuming foods like this are fine on occasion but not a good idea to have regularly, particularly if your goal is to lose weight.

Now, the fat category is broken down further into two sub-sections, *Saturated Fat* and *Trans-Fats*. Remember earlier when I talked about the chemical "hydrogenated vegetable oil"? Those are known as "trans-fats" and something the FDA has recently started recognizing as "not safe" in ANY amount. Tran-fats are directly linked to increased "bad" cholesterol and, in turn, heart disease. This is the reason why many countries have either already banned trans-fats or are moving closer to doing so. However, the bad news is that even if you see a product contains zero trans-fats on the label it could STILL legally contain up to .5g.

When it comes to *Saturated Fat*, a major contributor to obesity and heart disease, you should steer clear of these products as much as possible. Products likely to contain saturated or trans-fats are ones containing dairy, vegetable or seed oils.

Fiber - As I mentioned earlier, virtually all diseases are triggered by toxins entering the bloodstream through our intestinal lining. This is directly related to not getting enough fiber in our diet, which helps "sweep away" waste and detoxify our body. Fiber helps clean our bowels, aids digestion and prevents waste from sitting in our colon for too long.

How much fiber do we need? First, *think about how many bowel movements you have each day. If you aren't having at least one per day that is a clear sign you're not including enough fiber in your diet.* The ONLY foods containing fiber are plant-based, most notably beans/legumes, broccoli, artichokes, avocados, pears, raspberries, blackberries, sweet potatoes and certain grains such as brown rice. Begin eating more of these foods until you are having regular bowel movements.

When choosing a pre-packaged food, try selecting ones with the most fiber. Even if you're just buying something as simple as rice cakes, go with the one that has 1g of fiber as opposed to the one with zero fiber.

Cholesterol – There are two types of cholesterol, good (HDL) and bad (LDL). To keep it simple, know the "good" is the kind we make ourselves which our body uses to keep cells healthy. The "bad" kind is known as dietary cholesterol, which means taking in ADDITIONAL cholesterol from the foods we eat. The only foods containing cholesterol are ones derived from other living beings, or animal products. The human body is not very efficient at eliminating dietary cholesterol which is why the regular consumption of animal-based products can lead to someone having "high cholesterol" and, in some cases, to more serious conditions such as heart disease. Bad cholesterol aids in the formation of plaques in our arteries, leading to clogging and eventually, strokes or heart attacks. It's best to either limit or just remove animal-based cholesterol as much as possible in order to maintain optimal health. Remember earlier how I mentioned the USDA will not allow ANY company to claim eggs as "nutritious" or "healthy"? This is because they also know that even HALF an egg contains more cholesterol than we should be consuming on any regular basis. For this reason, try to only buy products indicating ZERO cholesterol.

LESS IMPORTANT

Below are the less important areas of the Nutrition Facts label because they tend to be centered on NUMBERS, as if you're keeping track of them, tallying between meals and trying to reach some magic amount by the end of the day. Doing so only results in confusion, frustration and eventually, giving up.

The only ones who really need to care about numbers would be athletes, wanting to know PRECISELY what they're consuming or perhaps someone with an extreme medical condition having to monitor their intake of certain ingredients, such as sodium or sugar. Otherwise, *it's more important for the average consumer to know the INGREDIENTS and have an understanding of CALORIES from FAT* than worry about exactly how much salt, sugar, carbohydrates or protein are in a particular food.

Carbohydrates – The number associated with "carbs" indicates how much energy you'll get from that food at the recommended serving size. For example, if you find a cereal with 40g of carbs, you know it will satisfy you LONGER than a cereal with 20g at the same serving size. Why? Remember, *carbohydrates give us ENERGY, the more the better.*

Sugar – The reason I didn't include this in the "most important" section above is because EVERY cell in our body needs sugar for fuel. Does this mean we should eat endless amounts of it, regardless of where it comes from? No.

If you're choosing products wisely by checking the ingredients list FIRST, this area is of less concern. You may remember from earlier that 1 gram of sugar equals 4 calories. So the problem with eating or drinking something high in sugar is not necessarily the sugar itself, but the CALORIES associated with it.

This is why soda drinkers would greatly benefit from ending this habit because each can is packed with around 40 grams of sugar, or 176 calories. If you drank only two cans of soda each day and stopped, you would reduce your daily caloric intake by over 350 calories! Don't forget, *we gain weight by consuming MORE calories than our body is burning off.* Therefore, anything you can do to reduce unnecessary calories, the better off you will be.

Sodium (Salt) – Like sugar, our taste buds are DESIGNED to detect and derive great satisfaction from salt. Did nature make a mistake or play a cruel joke on us so we are built to taste and enjoy salt, but have to avoid it? No.

Like sugar, salt can be consumed in less healthy ways. The problem with salt is that it's usually paired up with foods such as salami or cheese which are unhealthy for other reasons. However, salt itself is good for us and not something we should be overly concerned about, unless perhaps, we have an EXTRAORDINARY amount of it or have a serious health condition requiring a closer look at sodium intake.

Sprinkling a modest amount of salt onto a meal to taste is perfectly fine. I would suggest seeking out Pink Himalayan or Celtic Sea Salt as these are not refined like regular table salt and have retained a host of natural minerals, such as iodine, which helps detoxify our thyroid gland.

As a rule of thumb, try to keep the salt to calorie ratio at 1:1. Meaning, if something has 50 calories/serving, it should have no more than 50mg of sodium/serving. Optimally, we should max out around 1500 mg of salt per day. This doesn't mean you have to carry a calculator at all times and keep a "salt tally", just use this information as a GUIDE. For example, if you see a frozen pizza with 780 mg of salt per serving (1/4th of pie), this means if you eat just HALF the pie yourself you're consuming enough to meet your ENTIRE daily recommended amount. By the time your day is done and you've consumed other foods, you could have EASILY exceeded your daily salt intake by 10 times.

Protein – Considering sickness and disease due to protein deficiency is virtually unheard of in human history, it's safe to say we don't need to worry too much about protein numbers on the backs of packaged foods. Earlier I mentioned how the human body doesn't store excess protein and could be treated as TOXINS when consumed in large amounts. If you're eating mostly plant-based, WHOLE foods you will EASILY meet your daily protein requirements and be consuming them in the best possible way, with a host of other vitamins and minerals your body can use efficiently. In other words, the numbers associated with protein are nice to know, but not something you should be basing decisions on.

USELESS INFORMATION

On the nutritional facts label, you can disregard any of the "% of daily value" numbers. They are based on national guidelines that are not realistic and so convoluted you wouldn't understand how they arrived at those numbers in the first place. Also, don't pay attention to the vitamin content either. Are you really going to start keeping track of how much Vitamin A you had today? It's ridiculous to even begin caring about this type of information. If you're eating the right foods, you will EASILY reach and exceed any amounts required by your body to function normally.

IS EATING HEALTHY TOO EXPENSIVE?

One thing that scares people away from buying healthier or even certified organic is they think it's too expensive. While organic products are usually a little pricier than their conventional counterpart, you need to look at the bigger picture.

If you are really getting serious about eating healthier, you may start consuming less restaurant food, junk food and animal products than you normally buy. Most people buy enough meat and dairy for three meals a day, seven days a week. It's not uncommon to have sausage and eggs for breakfast, sandwich meat and cheese for lunch, maybe yogurt in the afternoon, perhaps steak, beef and chicken for dinner and likely more milk and dairy for dessert.

When you consider how much your health risks INCREASE on a steady diet of animal products, even if you can cut consumption down by a QUARTER, you would save enough money to accommodate the addition of organic products. Eventually reduce your consumption of animal products by 50%, and you will really start saving on your overall grocery bill.

Keep in mind; *starches are among the cheapest foods on the planet*. Rice, corn, beans and potatoes are all very inexpensive especially when bought in BULK.

Food	Price/lb.	Food	Price/lb.
Bacon	$4.53	Potatoes	$.80
Cheese	$4.25	Apples	$1.36
Beef	$3.70	Rice	$.69
Chicken	$3.17	Bananas	$.50
		Beans	$1.45
		Tomatoes	$1.12

(All prices are from the Friday, May 2, 2014 USDA's National Fruit and Vegetable Report, which is issued weekly.)

SECTION HIGHLIGHTS (Ch. 7)

- Healthy eating begins with what you put in your shopping cart because, ultimately, that's what you wind up bringing home and eating.

- Most of the products in any given grocery store are useless to a healthy diet.

- If you only change ONE thing about the way you're currently eating, you are on the right path.

- Products containing the USDA Certified Organic logo are held to an additional set of standards which go above and beyond those in conventional products.

- When buying certified organic, you're simply REDUCING health risks by consuming foods free of pesticides and artificial ingredients more than anything else.

- The only ones who really need to be concerned with gluten free foods are those suffering from a condition known as "celiac disease".

- Foods containing GMOs are not required by law to be labeled in the USA. Since companies involved with the manufacturing of GMO products don't consider our health a priority, it's best to steer clear of these products whenever possible.

- While not all packaged foods in America are unhealthy, around 80% of them contain ingredients that have been BANNED in other countries.

- Don't believe any claims made on the front of any packaged food product.

- Before examining the nutritional information, check to see what is actually exactly IN any given product. The longer the ingredients list, the more PROCESSING went into making the product.

- Make sure no more than 20% of the calories you're eating per serving come from fat.

- Try to buy foods that contain at least 1g of fiber per serving to maintain proper bowel function.

- As a rule of thumb, try to keep the salt to calorie ration at 1:1. Meaning, if something has 50 calories/serving, it should have no more than 50mg of sodium/serving.

- Starches are among the cheapest foods on the planet, especially when purchased in BULK.

CHAPTER EIGHT
Final Thoughts

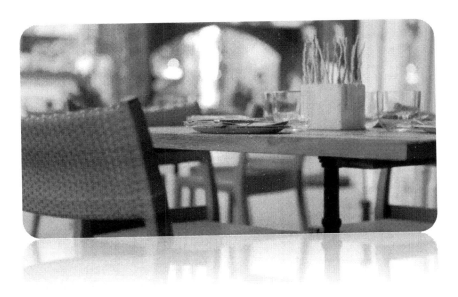

"In this book I have outlined the Top 5 steps ANYONE can take to DRAMATICALLY improve their health no matter what illness, disease or health condition they currently struggle with. Make no mistake; NOBODY can look out for your health more than YOU!"

FINAL THOUGHTS

I've used cars as an example many times throughout this book because, like cars, the better we take care of our "engines" the longer we can "drive" them. Ever known someone who bought a used car that was previously owned by an elderly person? In most cases, they're AMAZED at how these cars are kept in such exceptional condition. Why? They were used in MODERATION and not likely to have been pushed to their limits very often.

While writing this book I often thought about my grandmother, who recently turned 92 years of age. Not only is she in her early 90's, but she lives on her own, has a social life and is generally healthy. I asked her not too long ago how she did it – how has she managed to take such good care of herself?

For someone who was born in the early 1920's, she spent her childhood years living under "The Great Depression", where food consumption was guided more by how much you could afford than having the luxury of too many options. In those early years, most meals were centered around plant-based foods as meat was simply too expensive to consume on a daily basis. At that time, ALL food was produced closer to what we now call "certified organic" and not exposed to the same amounts of saturated fat, artificial flavors, chemicals, insecticides, pesticides, antibiotics and growth hormones that we see today.

By the time fast food restaurants or convenience foods became vastly popular she was already an adult with a family of her own. Because she was raised consuming healthier foods and eating in moderation, she continued this tradition throughout her entire adult life and it is, I believe, the primary reason she is still with us today and in such good health.

How far we have come…

While someone from my grandmother's generation may not have touched fast food until their adult years, nowadays it's almost expected that children in the United States begin their fast food journey as young as TWO years old. It's estimated we have finally reached a point in modern history where today's parents are predicted to actually OUTLIVE their own children. It simply doesn't have to be like this.

Stop for a moment and think about how you'd like to spend the final 15 years of your life. Would you like to spend them in sickness, slowly deteriorating to the point where you're simply not able to function at all? Do you want those final years to be spent with a loved one who has to take care of your EVERY need, or would you rather be in a position where you can fully enjoy sharing life with your family and friends, making the most of every day?

In this book I have outlined the Top 5 steps ANYONE can take to DRAMATICALLY improve their health no matter what illness, disease or health condition they currently struggle with. Make no mistake; *NOBODY can look out for your health more than YOU!*

Most people trust doctors with their lives. *While doctors mean well, most are never EDUCATED about the direct relation between diet and health.* When you consider a doctor's education is either provided or funded by the multi-billion dollar pharmaceutical industry, it should come as no surprise.

In my opinion, a responsible doctor today is one who looks at, understands and prescribes a change in DIET ahead of any prescription drug. If you are currently seeing a doctor, it's important to have them understand you are now more focused on DIET, with a goal of reducing your current medications and, ultimately, getting off them completely. It's important to work WITH your doctor so they can monitor your progress and address any adjustments in medication accordingly. If, for some reason, your doctor is not agreeable to this, it may be time to find another one who is. Your life depends on it.

SOMETHING YOU NEVER HEAR

Here's a conversation you NEVER hear in a doctor's office…

"Hey doc, I know cigarettes can cause lung cancer… so how many do you think I can smoke so it doesn't happen to me?"

How does a responsible doctor answer that kind of question? Of course they would recommend not smoking *at all.*

Now, here's a question for YOU…

Knowing that too much dietary cholesterol, animal protein, saturated fat and chemically-laden foods increases your likelihood of sickness, obesity, heart disease, diabetes or cancer… how much will you consume so it doesn't happen to you?

CHAPTER NINE
Food and Drink Ideas

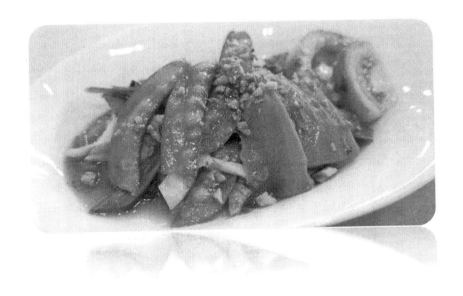

"The sources listed below are the result of two years' worth of research, application and personal growth. What began as a journey of self-improvement has become a mission to share what I've learned with you, the reader."

PLANT-BASED, WHOLE FOOD MEAL IDEAS...

Breakfast

- Whole Fruit (banana, apple, grapes, blueberries, strawberries, peaches, pear, etc.)
- Bowl of Oatmeal (whole grain rolled oats with cinnamon, raisins, fruits, honey)
- Cereal Bowl w/fruit and nut milk. (Uncle Sam Cereal, shredded wheat, USDA organic low-fat varieties)
- Green or Fruit Smoothie
- Whole Grain Bagel or Toast with nut butter or jelly.
- Whole grain pancakes/waffles with organic maple syrup

Lunch

- Salad (with lettuce, spinach, tomato, carrots, cucumber, avocado, olives or walnuts)
- Soups (tomato basil, lentil, vegetable, split pea, potato)
- Hash Browns (light oil to coat or use a non-stick pan)
- Baked Potato (white or sweet) w/gravy (non-dairy)
- Whole Fruit (banana, apple, grapes, blueberries, strawberries, peaches, pear, etc.)
- Sandwich with homemade hummus, tomato and lettuce on whole grain bread
- Wraps or Pitas (with beans, tomato, mushrooms, corn, lettuce, onions or hummus)

Dinner

- White or Sweet Potatoes (mashed, baked, steamed, wedges, fries, rounds, hash browns)
- Bean Burrito, Enchiladas or Tacos w/refried beans, rice, corn, salsa.
- Rice (white or brown) w/black beans, tofu or tempeh
- Pasta w/marinara, pesto sauce
- Stir-Fry (vegetables, rice, Asian noodles, curry, tofu)
- Vegetables such as green beans, carrots, corn, roasted bell peppers or asparagus.
- Burgers (veggie, bean, Portobello mushroom)

Snacks

- Green or Fruit Smoothie
- Whole Fruit or Bowl (banana, apple, grapes, blueberries, strawberries, peaches, pear, etc.)
- Nuts (handful)
- Peanut Butter and Jelly sandwich on whole grain bread.
- Corn Chips (low fat) with beans, tomatoes, guacamole, lettuce or salsa)
- Air-popped Popcorn (flavored with salt/nutritional yeast, onion powder, paprika, etc.)
- Potato wedges/fries (Sweet or White with organic ketchup or custom dip – olive oil not needed.)
- Kale Chips
- Whole grain bread w/nut butter or hummus.
- Veggies (carrots/celery/broccoli) with dip (hummus, nut butter)

Recommended Beverages

- **100% Spring Water (at least 5 glasses/day)**
- **Carbonated water with a light amount of fruit juice from concentrate to taste.**
- **Green tea, hibiscus tea, ginger tea**
- **Organic nut milks (almond, coconut, hemp, rice, soy)**

My Personal Favorite Brands *

- **Dave's Killer Bread (my favorite bread, hands down!)**
- **Ezekiel 4:9 (bread, muffins, tortillas and more)**
- **365 Organic (Whole Foods brand)**
- **Simple Truth Organic (Kroger brand)**
- **Engine 2 Plant-Strong (Rip Esselstyn)**
- **Navitas Naturals (cacao, maca, gogi berries, etc.)**
- **Healthworks (cacao, maca, gogi berries, etc.)**
- **Uncle Sam (cereal)**
- **Cascadia Farm (cereal)**
- **Silk (nut/plant milks)**
- **Lightlife (tempeh)**
- **Sweet Earth (seitan, veggie burgers, etc.)**
- **Muir Glen Organic (pasta sauce)**
- **Eat Barbeque (BBQ sauce)**
- **Mrs. Dash (salt-free, delicious seasonings)**

* NOTE: While I endorse the above brands and find most of their products excellent choices, ALWAYS read the ingredients first on <u>any</u> product to see if it supports healthy guidelines. And remember, the absolute healthiest foods (pulled from the Earth) do not carry a brand or label.

FIVE EASY RECIPES

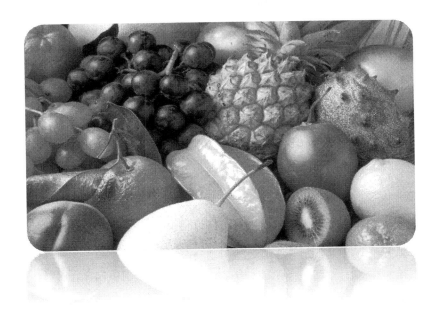

Here are five easy and healthy plant-based recipes that are among my personal favorites!

I Can't Believe It's Not Pudding!

- 1 avocado (peeled and pitted)
- ¼ cup raw Cacao Powder
- 2-3 tbsp. agave nectar (or raw honey)
- ½ tsp. vanilla extract
- ½ cup soy milk (unsweetened)

How To:

- Add all of the above ingredients to a blender or food processor
- Blend until mixture is creamy smooth
- Refrigerate for at least two hours and then serve.

Comments: Friends will be amazed to learn how avocado powers this delicious and healthy snack.

Healthy Hummus

- 1 can garbanzo/chick beans (15oz can)
- 1 can cannellini beans (15oz can)
- 2 cloves of garlic (large)
- 1 lemon (juiced)
- 1 tsp. cumin powder
- 1 tsp. sea salt
- ¼ tsp. white pepper
- 2 tbsp. tahini (no added oil)
- ¼ - ½ drained liquid from canned beans

How To:

- Add all of the above ingredients to a blender or food processor
- Blend until desired texture
- Serve immediately.

Comments: Add more/less liquid depending on how thick/runny you prefer the hummus. Great to serve with pita bread or spread on whole grain bread.

BBQ Tempeh Burritos

- ½ block of tempeh (4oz., organic)
- ¼ leaf of Kale
- 1 cup cooked rice (white or brown)
- Pumpkin Seeds (small handful)
- BBQ Sauce (organic or w/o artificial ingredients, or high fructose corn syrup)
- 1 Avocado (optional)
- 2 Tortillas (organic flour, corn, whole grain)

How To:

- Boil half block (4oz.) of tempeh for 15-20 minutes.
- Chop tempeh into strips, lightly coat skillet on medium heat with coconut oil so as not to stick, cook until golden brown on both sides, reduce heat to low, toss in BBQ sauce and stir to thoroughly coat tempeh, cover skillet until ready to serve.
- On another skillet, lightly brown both sides of each tortilla.
- Lay down kale on tortilla

- Add cooked rice
- Add avocado slice (optional)
- Add strips of tempeh (3-4)
- Add Pumpkin seeds on top
- Roll burritos (2) and serve

Comments: Very important to boil the tempeh and remove the bitterness. Look for organic tortillas in the frozen section of Whole Foods or other health food stores. Experiment with other ingredients to add more flavors! A great way to eat extra leftovers too.

Friendly Fries

- 1 large Russet potato (skin on)
- Your favorite seasonings
- Ketchup (organic)
- Parchment paper

How To:

- Preheat oven to 400F
- Chop potato in half vertically and then halve it again. Chop potato into ½ strips (wedges)
- Add potato to mixing bowl, add in your favorite seasonings and gently toss until wedges are fully coated.
- Add potatoes to cookie sheet lined with parchment paper.
- Cook at 400F for 25-30 minutes.
- Once done, serve with ketchup

Comments: Be sure the wedges are fairly equal in size so they cook evenly. Serve with ketchup or your favorite condiment. Great with garlic, onion, paprika, sea salt and nutritional yeast, among others.

Easy As Pumpkin Pie

- 1 can pumpkin (15oz, organic)
- 1 cup non-dairy milk
- 1 tsp. vanilla extract
- ½ cup agave nectar (or 3/4 cup of sugar)
- 1 tbsp. apple cider vinegar
- ¼ cup all-purpose flower
- 1 tsp. baking powder
- ½ tsp. sea salt
- 1 tsp. cinnamon
- ¾ tsp. ginger
- ½ tsp. nutmeg
- Whole wheat pie crust (organic)

How To:

- Preheat oven to 375F
- Add above ingredients into a mixing bowl and mix well.
- Pour into pie crust and smooth evenly
- Cook at 375F for 45 minutes.
- Allow pie to cool for 20 minutes, then either serve hot or refrigerate.

Comments: A great, easy to make, healthy snack anytime, especially with coffee after dinner.

REFERENCES

The sources listed below are the result of years' worth of research, application and personal growth. What began as a journey of self-improvement has become a mission to share what I've learned with you, the reader. Many of the people listed below have changed my life for the better and I can't thank them enough for their insights and inspiration: (listed in alphabetical order)

Abby Martin
ABC News
About.com
Active.com
AuthorityNutrition.com
Babble.com
BlacklistedNews.com
Care2.com
CDC.gov
CinnamonVogue.com
CNN.com
Coast To Coast Am (12/23/13) George Noory w/John McDougall
ConsumerReports.org
Corinna Rachel w/Gwen Olsen, "Why We Can't Trust Our Doctors: Ex-Pharma Drug Rep Tells All" (interview)
Cowspiracy (film)
CSPInet.org
Dairy.org
Dani Spies (YouTube)
Doug Lisle, Ph.D., "Lose Weight Without Losing Your Mind" (lecture)
Dr. Caldwell Esselstyn
Dr. Denis Burkitt
Dr. Edward Group, "The Green Body Cleanse" (book)
Dr. Garth Davis, "Proteinaholic" (book)
Dr. Kathleen DesMaisons, "Potatoes Not Prozac" (book)
Dr. Michael Greger "How Not To Die" (book), lectures
Dr. Michael Klaper
Dr. Neal Barnard

DrMcDougall.com (website and YouTube)
Earthlings (film)
ECFR.gov
ExcuseProof.com
FDA.gov
FedUp (film)
Finance.Yahoo.com
Food52.com
FoodBabe.com (Vani Hari), "The Food Babe Way" (book)
FoodMatters.tv
Forks Over Knives (film)
Freelee & Harley (30BananasaDay.com)
GMOAnswers.com
GMOFreeUSA.org
Happy Healthy Vegan (YouTube)
Health.Harvard.Edu
HuffingtonPost.com
Hungry For Change (film)
Jane Moore "Supermarket Secrets & Deceptions" (documentary)
Jeff Novick, R.D., M.S.
Joe Cross (RebootWithJoe.com, "Fat Sick & Nearly Dead" (film)
John Kohler (DiscountJuicers.com)
John McDougall, MD "The Starch Solution" (book and lectures)
John Westerdahl, Ph.D. "The Power of Plant Foods in Anti-Aging
  and Lifestyle Medicine" (lecture)
LabelWatch.com
Livestrong.com
LivingMaxwell.com
LLS.org
Lunch Hour (film)
Mark Sisson. "The Primal Blueprint" (book)
MedicineNet.com
Michael Moss, "Salt Sugar Fat" (book)
Michael Pollan, "Food Rules" (book)
Michael Tapp
Mike Adams, Health Ranger
Milton Mills, M.D. "Are Humans Designed To Eat Meat?" (lecture)
MindBodyGreen.com

MSGTruth.org
NaturalNews.com
New York Times
Nomad Man Productions and the Benner Family Homestead,
  "Today's Modern Food, it's Not What You Think" (documentary)
NonGMOProject.org
NPR.org
Nutribullet
NutritionFacts.org
Nutrition.McDonalds.com
PCRM.org
Potato Strong (YouTube)
Prevention.com
RawFamily.com
Rip Esselstyn – "The Engine 2 Diet" (book) and TedEx lecture
Rodale News
RootsNatural.ca
T. Colin Campbell Ph.D, "The China Study" and "Whole" (book)
TakePart.com
ThinkProgress.org
UndergoundHealth.com
US National Library of Medicine/National Institutes of Health
USDA.gov
USDA-FDA.com
VegSource.com
Vitamix
WakingTimes.com
Wall Street Journal
WebMD.com

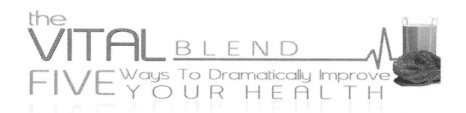

A very special THANK YOU to the family and friends, who have supported, engaged, challenged and inspired me for the past three years on this project.

Please visit our Web site at TheVitalBlend.com and follow us on Facebook.

www.TheVitalBlend.com

Book design by **ThatDesignChick.com.** Have a project of your own you'd like to explore? Email **info@ThatDesignChick.com** for a Solutions Advisor to help with Creative Consulting, Marketing, Branding or Graphic Design needs.

Made in the USA
Las Vegas, NV
02 March 2022